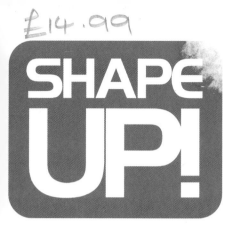

TAILOR-MADE TRAINING FOR
FEMALE BODY
SHAPES

CAROLINE SANDRY

AND JOHN SHEPHERD

A & C BLACK • LONDON

First published in 2008 by
A&C Black Publishers Ltd
38 Soho Square, London W1D 3HB
www.acblack.com

Copyright © Caroline Sandry and John Shepherd

ISBN 978 1 4081 0600 6

A CIP catalogue record for this book is available from the British Library.

Acknowledgements
Cover image © John Shepherd
Inside photography © Grant Pritchard, except p.103 © istock.com;
Illustrations p. 3 © Jeff Edwards; p. 40 Mark Silver and icons used throughout
by James Watson using images from istockphoto.com
Thanks to Patrick Dale, James Conaghan and Jacqui Ball of Solar Fitness, Cyprus,
for modelling and assisting with the organisation of the photo shoot. Solar Fitness
runs personal trainer and fitness instructor courses on the island – for further
information see www.solarfitness.com.

> **Note**
> Whilst every effort has been made to ensure the content of this book is as
> technically accurate as possible, neither the authors nor the publishers can
> accept responsibility for any injury or loss sustained as a result of the use of
> this material.

Many thanks also to USA Pro for supplying the outfits used in the photo shoot.
This book is produced using paper that is made from wood grown in managed,
sustainable forests. It is natural, renewable and recyclable. The logging and
manufacturing processes conform to the environmental regulations of the country
of origin.

Typeset in URWGrotesk by Palimpsest Book Production Limited, Grangemouth,
Stirlingshire

Printed and bound in China by South China Printing Co.

CONTENTS

ACKNOWLEDGEMENTS

I would firstly like to thank John Shepherd for believing in me, and giving me the chance to write this book, and secondly A&C Black – most notably Lucy Beevor for her patience and support.

I would like to dedicate this book to all my training clients, and class members who are so loyal and all feel like friends to me. These people are more important in terms of learning and experience than anything, and are so kind in supporting me through all of my work projects. Thank you!

Thank you to my wonderful friends Viki Harvey and Lucy Gardner for their time, energy and support.

Last but not least, I would like top thank Grant Pritchard our genius photographer, and Pat, Jim, Vicky and Jacqui at Solar Fitness for their help in Cyprus.

FOREWORD

Over the past few years, whenever I have needed to lose weight or improve my fitness for a project, such as for my roles in *Chicago* and *Guys and Dolls*, I have trained with Caroline Sandry and achieved great results.

I have the disadvantage of having a bad back, but through incorporating Pilates into our training sessions, I have strengthened my back while losing weight and toning up.

I am typically a pear shape, and had always found it hard to lose inches from my hips and thighs. However, using Caroline's tailor-made programmes my body shape really changed. In the past I have sweated it out in the gym, doing countless repetitions of exercises that I didn't enjoy and I never felt as if the results I gained matched the effort I put in. However, Caroline and I trained mostly outside, which I loved, and the exercises were much more focused and concentrated, meaning less repetitions with better results. Perfect! My figure is now longer and leaner and I have the knowledge to keep it that way.

Good luck with your training!

Claire Sweeney
Actress, singer, presenter

INTRODUCTION

Whether you have skinny arms and a big bottom, or wide hips and a flat stomach, whether you are slim or not so slim, this book will show you how to look your best.

Many women are unhappy with their body image. In today's celebrity-obsessed culture, we are being bombarded with images of perfectly proportioned bodies and flawless faces, making us increasingly negative about our own appearance. As a model in my younger years, I succumbed to this pressure, and tried a variety of diets that were not only boring, but also pretty unhealthy. A restricted calorie intake generally produces lethargy – not what is required to be fit and healthy! And if you restrict your food intake enough, you can actually end up heavier than before you started (more about that later).

So how realistic are these images we are sold every day? Actually, very unrealistic! It has been known for fashion magazines and advertising campaigns to take an already beautiful model, and then digitally stretch her legs to make them impossibly long and lean, air-brush her stomach until it's as flat as a pancake, and correct any minor imperfections to create a perfect specimen to sell their product – I speak from experience!

I have always loved exercise and fitness. I used to cycle and horse-ride when I was at school, but I didn't discover the gym until my twenties, and that was when I acknowledged my passion for fitness. I am now lucky enough to make a living out of training women (and men) of all shapes and sizes, and I have learnt an enormous amount from their experiences.

In writing this book, I hope to give you the dietary and fitness facts that will help you make the very most of yourself. I have included sections on resistance and cardiovascular training, and simple programmes to follow. I will explain which exercises and programmes *will* work for 'your' body, and not some idealised standard. You will discover all the information you need to achieve your goals, whatever your age, sports or fitness level, safely, quickly and effectively. None of us are perfect, but we can all improve what we have been given.

Caroline Sandry

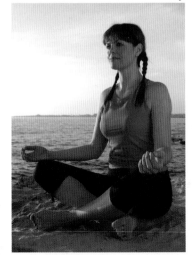

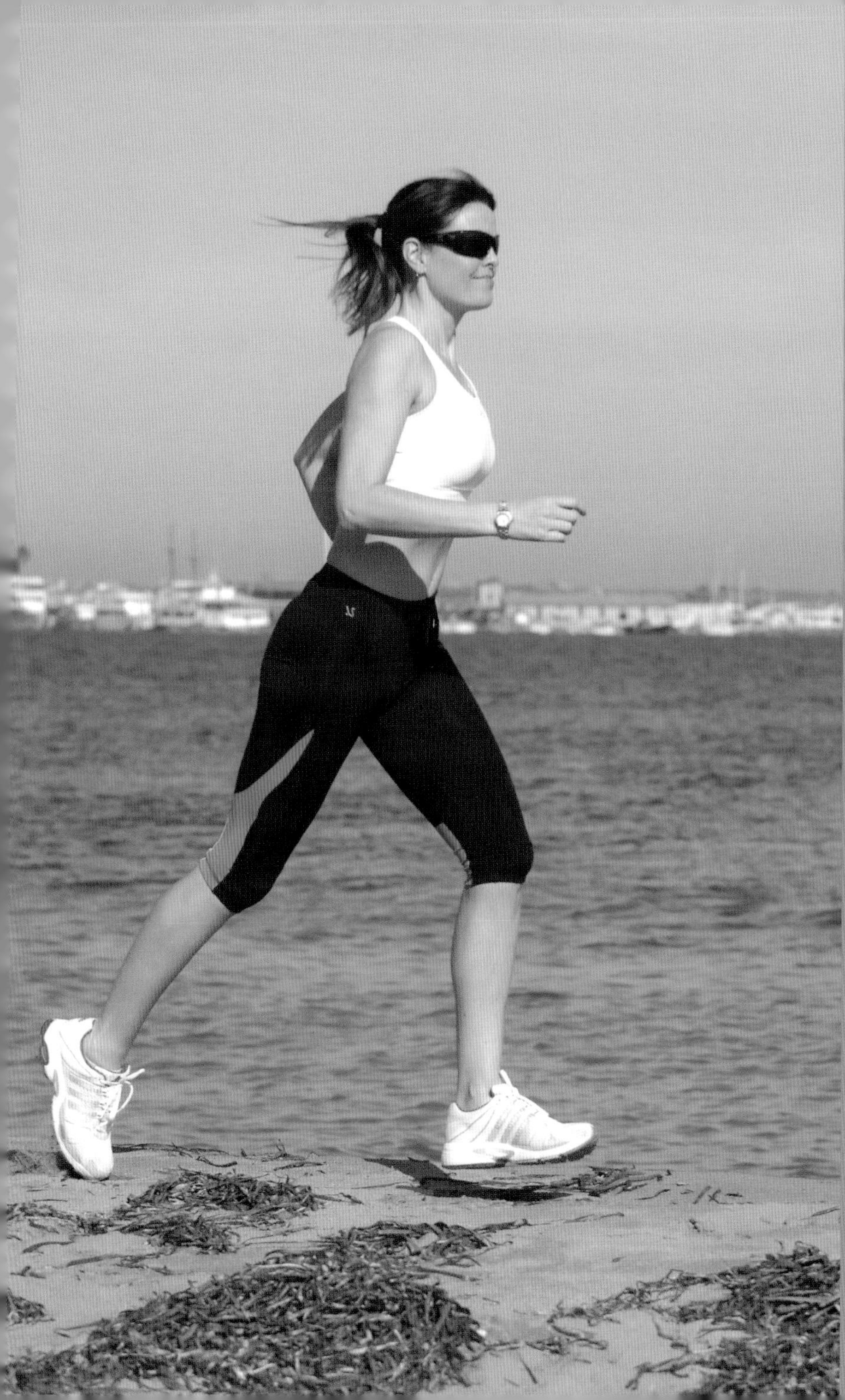

1 UNDERSTANDING YOUR BODY AND KNOWING YOUR BODY TYPE

Do you wish you had long slim legs like Elle McPherson or that you were slim and petite like Kylie Minogue? Well, unfortunately if you crave Kylie, but look more like Geraldine, the Vicar of Dibley, then the harsh truth is that your wishes are wasted! We all have our body 'blueprint' set at an early age, and there are limits to how much change we can create.

There are three basic body types. The mesomorph is a generally athletic body type, with a narrow waist, broad shoulders and long limbs; this type will easily gain muscle and tends to be naturally sporty. The ectomorph is slimmer with a smaller body frame, tends to have lower body fat, and can find it hard to gain weight. The endomorph is rounder and larger and will tend to store body fat, so can gain weight easily. Most of us will have a combination of elements from more than one body type, but be predominately one. The information in this book will help you to maximise your shape, tone, strength and fitness whatever your body type.

In Part 1 of the book I'll provide you with the information needed to identify your body type. I'll also provide an overview of the key aspects of female physiology – how we respond to exercise. Understanding this will make it much easier to relate to and use the information provided in the practical training sections – for example, understanding the importance of resistance (weight) training and how it will positively affect your metabolism, leading to increased calorie burning. I also provide some health-related information – notably on body weight, fat levels and obesity. These are presented to indicate just why embarking on a fitness programme that reflects your body type could be the most important thing you've ever done for yourself.

What's your body type?

As I've indicated, there are three main body types (or, more specifically, 'somatotypes') – these are ectomorphs, mesomorphs and endomorphs. This basic classification dates back to the mid-twentieth century, when the psychologist William Sheldon identified three different body shapes – basically 'fat', 'thin' and 'athletic'. He believed that each somatotype had distinct physiological (and psychological) traits, and although his work is maybe overstated, it provides a highly valuable starting point for the analysis of body types because it helps us to identify the ways that these will typically respond physiologically to training.

Use Table 1 to identify your body type. Remember – you will probably be a mix of two or even three types, but predominately one main somatotype. I need to point out now that your body type is different from your body shape (*see* page 6). You should also use the Body Mass Index (BMI) on page 8 to identify whether you are underweight, of ideal weight or overweight.

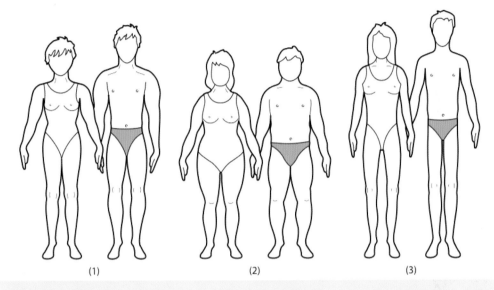

Fig. 1.1 *The three main body types: (1) Ectomorph (2) Mesomorph (3) Endomorph*

The difference between body type and body shape – 'nature versus nurture'

I am guessing that you bought this book because you would like to improve your body shape. Perhaps you have lost what 'mother nature' gave you and you're now overweight. You might think that doing athletics or even going for a light jog is beyond you, but with the right training programme, and understanding your body type, you can make significant changes.

As we have noted, your body type is what mother nature predetermined at an early age (nature). If you think back to your adolescence, you will have a pretty good idea of your soma-totype. Your body shape, however, is more changeable and is the result of your everyday life, training and diet (nurture). Take, for example, a mesomorphic-type female long-distance runner. Due to her long periods of intense training, she may develop a more ecto-morphic body shape. Or take a mesomorphic woman who leads a sedentary lifestyle and

---

TABLE 1 Different body types and their characteristics

Mesomorphs

BODY CHARACTERISTICS
- Usually tall with broad shoulders and a narrow waist ■ Athletic build ■ Strong arms and legs ■ Upright posture ■ Good muscular definition ■ Have fairly fast metabolism

FITNESS/SPORTS ADVANTAGES/SUITABILITY
- Mesomorphs respond well to CV and resistance training, due to their adaptable and responsive physiology ■ They can sustain low body-fat levels ■ Dependent on fitness/sports needs, they will find it relatively easy to gain or lose weight ■ Can be freer with their food choices – but this does not mean eating unhealthily

FITNESS/SPORTS DISADVANTAGES
- Mesomorphs can over-train (*see* page 114), as their bodies are quite robust when it comes to training. They should therefore try to keep balance in their training and be mindful that higher-intensity work must be moderated. Yoga and Pilates help create balance ■ They can put on weight quickly when they stop training ■ Their training needs to be progressive and constantly changing to prevent stagnation. This results from their ability to respond more quickly than the other two body types to training

Ectomorph

BODY CHARACTERISTICS
- Slight frame with low body-fat levels ■ Medium to tall height, long limbs and thin face ■ Fast metabolism – hence crucial need to *increase* calorie consumption to build muscle and add curves and maintain training readiness – they need to create a 'positive energy balance' (*see* page 122)

Ectomorph (cont.)

FITNESS/SPORTS ADVANTAGES/SUITABILITY
■ Light frame makes them suited for aerobic activity ■ Additionally smaller body surface area enhances their suitability for endurance activity, as their bodies are better at keeping cool

FITNESS/SPORTS DISA.DVANTAGES
■ Can achieve low body-fat levels, which can be detrimental to health and hormones ■ Can find it difficult to build muscle mass if participating in a sport that benefits from this or for aesthetic reasons ■ Can be more prone to injury, therefore need to follow a rigorous pre-conditioning programme (*see* page 37)

Endomorphs

BODY CHARACTERISTICS
■ Have large frames, with a 'strong' appearance ■ Unfortunately this can come with a high body fat percentage, with fat being stored around the waist, hips and thighs ■ Medium to tall ■ Fairly slow metabolism

FITNESS/SPORTS ADVANTAGES/SUITABILITY
■ Shape benefits sports such as rugby and shot putting where size can be useful as long as it can be moved powerfully ■ Often have large lung capacities which can make them suited to, for example, rowing (*see* page 27) ■ Can increase strength much more easily than ectomorphs

FITNESS/SPORTS DISADVANTAGES
■ Their weight can make it difficult to perform sustained aerobic activity such as running, due to the impact forces involved and the stress this can place on joints ■ Can gain weight easily and lose condition quickly if training is ceased and calorie control not followed

eats a high-calorie/high-fat diet – she will develop an endomorphic body shape. With levels of obesity rising like never before, millions of women (and men) are taking on a more endomorphic shape due to lack of exercise and excess food consumption.

Training tip

Although two women may have the same body type, this does not mean that they'll respond to training in the same way. Each one of us will need to find the specific blend of training that works for us.

What's your body shape?

So, you have identified your body type, although it might have taken some memory recall to find it! Let's now establish your body shape using Table 2 opposite. I use icons to make it easier to identify just what your shape is.

Now you know your shape, it's time to shape up!

Having identified your existing body shape, we can get to work on using diet, lifestyle and exercise to make the best of your assets, and to work on your problem areas. Throughout the book, you will see the symbol for your body shape (apple, pear, etc.) to help you identify key points for your shape.

It is important to note that no two bodies are the same, and no two bodies will respond in an identical fashion to training and/or diet. It is also important to realise that even women with the most enviable figures should make fitness a part of their lives, as beauty and fitness is more than skin deep.

Obesity and female health problems

Obesity brings with it numerous potential health problems, such as osteoarthritis, heart disease, type 2 diabetes, high blood pressure, varicose veins, depression and even certain cancers (breast, uterus and colon). It has been calculated that this results in 30,000 deaths a year in the UK and a total cost to the country of £2 billion.

To find out if you are obese, underweight or overweight, take a look at the body mass index on page 8.

BODY MASS INDEX

Body Mass Index (or BMI) is used to estimate body composition and is calculated by dividing your weight in kilograms by the square of your height in metres.

BMI = weight (kg)/height (m^2)

Table 2 What's your body shape?			
Apple	**Pear**	**Hourglass**	**Celery**
Tend to carry weight around abdomen	Weight is stored on hips, bottom and thighs	Shoulders and hips are similar width	Shoulders, waist and hips are similar width
Bottom is small and flat	Often have slim waist and flat stomach	Curvy figure with full chest, but in proportion	Tend to have 'straight up and down' appearance, with narrow hips
Can have quite delicate wrists and ankles	Typically narrow shoulders	Tends to lose and gain weight evenly	Can be perceived as boyish, due to lack of curves
Best feature – slimmer hips and good legs	Best feature – nicely defined back and slim arms	Best feature – shapely waist	Best feature – often with sexy, long lean legs
Generous chest, can be out of proportion	Tend to lose weight from face and upper body	Bottom and hips may appear wide	Tends to lose weight evenly
Large chest and stomach can give 'barrel' appearance	Often has appearance of rounded shoulders	Upper arms may become fleshy	Chest tends to be relatively flat

What's my BMI?
- Underweight = <18.5
- Normal weight = 18.5–24.9
- Overweight = 25–29.9
- Obesity = BMI of 30 or greater

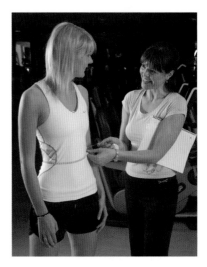

If your BMI is in excess of 35, you should contact your doctor.

There are limitations with BMI calculations, which can overestimate body fat in very muscular people and can underestimate it in people who have lost muscle mass (for example, the elderly). Also, if you are less than 5 feet tall you may not get an accurate BMI, due to anomalies with the calculation.

WAIST MEASUREMENT

Simply measuring your waist (around the belly button) can be a very good predictor of the health risks associated with obesity. If your measurement is in excess of 90cm (35.5 inches), you are at high risk, and if you measure in excess of 109cm (43.5 inches), you are at very high risk.

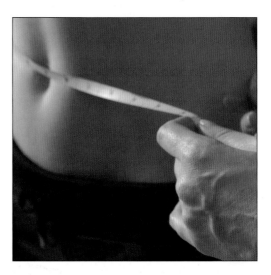

Cutting to the fat

As our levels of obesity rise, so too does our obsession with being slim. The media has an unhealthy obsession with celebrity bodies. This (unfortunately) sells scores of magazines – by headlining the actress with fat on her thighs, or the latest skinny 'size zero' celebrity. We are constantly being sold faddy 'get thin quick' diets and are bombarded with adverts for surgical procedures to cheat our way to perfection. Yet in spite of this current obsession for a slim physique, we are fatter than ever, and around 6 out of 10 of us will be overweight. So, what exactly is fat?

Fat is a source of energy, and it's one of the three macro-nutrients, along with protein and carbohydrate (*see* page 123). Fat is calorie dense when compared to the other macro-nutrients – containing about twice as many calories per gram (9 versus 4). What's not used for energy is stored in our bodies in various ways. Women tend to store body fat in different ways to men, and you are right when you lament to your partner 'but it's so much easier for men!' because women are genetically predisposed to having higher fat levels than men – this is why the pear shape is seen as a typical female body shape. We were programmed to store our fat around the hips and thighs in order to nourish and provide for a baby, even if food was scarce! To check healthy fat percentages, check fat guidelines on page 128.

Body composition

Our bodies are made up of different types of tissue: lean body tissue and adipose (fat) tissue.

LEAN BODY TISSUE (FAT-FREE MASS)

Lean body tissue is made up of muscles, bones, blood and organs. This tissue is metabolically active, meaning that it requires and uses energy to function. That's why increasing your lean mass through weights and other resistance training can contribute to increased calorie burning each and every day, even with your feet up.

More information on fat as a nutritional source can be found on page 128.

FAT (OR ADIPOSE) TISSUE

This tissue is made up of the following components:

- Essential fat: this is stored in bone marrow, the heart, lungs and liver and other vital organs; it supports life.
- Storage fat: this acts rather like a cushion, protecting the body's vital organs. It is spread around the body below the skin's surface (also known as subcutaneous fat).
- Non-essential fat: non-essential fat is just that; it's what makes us overweight and obese. It does not significantly fuel the body with energy (carbohydrate is the body's preferred activity fuel). It has no real purpose and is of course detrimental to our health if we store too much of it.

Body-fat testing

A body-fat (or body-composition) test can tell us whether our bodies have too much non-essential fat and what our lean (mainly muscle) weight is. There are various ways to measure body fat – for example, with bio-electrical impedance machines, callipers and calculations or even underwater weighing. However, most of us will be able to tell if we are carrying too much non-essential fat simply by looking at our bodies. However, I would suggest that you do not focus too much on your body fat – your fitness level is far more important. And if you do want to see how you are shaping up, use a good old-fashioned tape measure. This way you can gauge exactly where the changes are happening. A client of mine was recently most upset when five weeks into her programme, the scales did not show a significant weight loss; however, she was delighted when the tape measure showed she had actually lost 5.5 inches from her waist! Such a state of affairs resulted from the fact that muscle weighs more than fat. My client's body composition had altered positively; she had gained in lean weight and lost fat, but the scales did not show this.

If you do measure your own body fat, then anywhere between 20 per cent and 32 per cent is satisfactory for women's health. Body-fat levels below 20 per cent might be seen, for example, in healthy athletes, but in general fat levels below this range are not healthy and can lead to certain health problems (*see* page 11, being underweight).

FAT CELLS

The body has billions of fat cells. These can become larger (fat cell hypertrophy) or can increase in number (fat cell hyperplasia) through lack of exercise or poor dietary control.

> ### Training tip
>
> In terms of training to change your body shape you should focus on the outcomes of your training: the fact that your CV fitness is improving or that you are getting stronger or faster, rather than focusing on how much body fat you have. It's a given that if your fitness improves, so too will your body composition and shape.

HOW MANY FAT CELLS DO WE HAVE?

Non-obese	25–30 billion
Moderately obese	60–100 billion
Massively obese	300 billion

Up until quite recently it was thought that 'killing off' fat cells through working out and calorie controlled eating was impossible, but now exercise scientists believe we can get rid of fat cells permanently through a consistent exercise and dietary regime.

CELLULITE

Cellulite is just another type of fat. It's actually a term coined by the cosmetics industry that refers to that undesirable 'orange peel' look on skin. Forget the lotions and potions, combine weights and cardio at the gym. The CV exercise will burn calories and reduce excess body fat, while the resistance exercises will develop tone, definition, power and strength (in your legs and all over your body) and boost your metabolic rate by increasing your lean muscle mass. The right diet will also contribute to lean, toned thighs.

BEING UNDERWEIGHT

We have already noted that female athletes may have a very low body-fat percentage – take, for example, the amazing Paula Radcliffe, who has an incredibly lean physique due to her intense training and the need for a low body weight. Many ectomorphs (like Paula) may also have naturally low body-fat levels and could become underweight if they train without adjusting their calorie intake.

Being underweight can have serious implications for women, though, and this is why the trend for 'size zero' is so alarming. Being underweight cannot only affect your menstrual cycle, causing amenorrhoea (lack of menstruation), but it can impair your fertility and cause loss of libido (sex drive). Being underweight can also have an impact on your bone density, and can lead to osteoporosis (brittle bone disease).

You'll more than likely find that the restricted calorie intake also restricts nutrient intake – many women are iron deficient in the first place, and then increase their deficit by not eating enough. Someone who severely restricts her food, and/or trains excessively for weight loss, may also be suffering from an eating disorder.

Eating disorders in women

Eating disorders such as anorexia and bulimia are on the rise; an eating disorder is defined as 'having an obsessive interest in food and calories'.

Anorexia is a fear of fatness that goes way beyond that of most dieters. The need to control their weight dominates all other emotions in anorexics, and sufferers will go to great lengths – including excessive exercise, drastic calorie restriction, and the use of laxatives and vomiting – to lose weight.

Bulimia, like anorexia, starts with a compulsion to be thin, and involves bingeing on large quantities of food, followed by purging through vomiting and the use of laxatives.

THE BIOLOGICAL AND PSYCHOLOGICAL REASONS FOR EATING DISORDERS

There is no single cause for an eating disorder. It is a complex condition, probably caused by a variety of factors; these may include:

- Social pressure to be thin and sexually attractive.
- Genetics – those with a family history of anorexia may be more at risk of developing an eating disorder.
- Family relationships – parents of anorexics may be high achievers with too high expectations for their children, thus creating anxiety.
- Difficult life experiences such as bullying, abuse or bereavement, again creating anxiety that manifests itself in an eating disorder.
- Jobs that highlight body shape – for example, models or dancers may be more at risk. The same applies to certain sportswomen, such as gymnasts.

Anorexia and bulimia are psychiatric illnesses with specifically diagnosed traits. However, doctors have also defined 'sub-clinical eating disorders'. These are manifest in people who display some of the traits of the two eating disorders; these may be detrimental to health and need addressing. Such traits are particularly likely to be found in sports and fitness participants or those 'obsessed' with their appearance. This is because these people are often subject to great external pressure to conform to a certain body shape and look. They may also become convinced that less weight and ridiculously low body-fat levels will bring them success.

EATING DISORDER WARNING SIGNS

- Preoccupation with food and calories.
- Feeling and expressing that you are fat when you are not.
- Indications (or smells) of vomit in the bathroom.
- Mood swings.
- Excess use of laxatives.
- Secret eating.
- Unwillingness to eat in front of others.
- Large weight swings in a short space of time.

Be positive about your body shape

Research indicates that female athletes are highly at risk of suffering from eating disorders. One Spanish study focused on 283 elite sportswomen from numerous sports. It was discovered that 20 per cent of the women probably suffered from bulimia. This was five times greater than the Spanish average. Skaters and gymnasts were particularly likely to suffer from eating disorders, with 6 per cent fitting anorexia criteria.

It was argued that pressure from coaches was a big factor in how the women viewed their relationship with food. Coaches, it was found, often added to the negative feelings already felt by the women about their bodies.

Training tip

Avoiding sports- and fitness-related eating disorders

1 Have your dietary needs assessed by a nutrition expert. Research shows that those who control their own eating habits unsupervised are more likely to develop some kind of eating disorder.
2 Work with personal trainers and sports coaches who do not put unrealistic pressure on you to conform to a certain body shape or achieve unhealthily low body-fat levels.
3 Increase calorie consumption commensurately with increases in training volume.
4 If injured or ill, don't significantly reduce calorie consumption because you are not training. If you do this, you may not get all the nutrients you need to repair your injury or recover from your illness. Take expert advice.
5 Choose a fitness or sports activity that reflects your body type/current body shape. Doing this will prevent a possible 'mismatch' between your training and your aspirations for your body. To give an example, it would be unrealistic for an endomorph to achieve the slight frame of a distance runner.

We must all be mindful of the external pressures put on us to 'conform' to a certain body shape, whatever our sporting or fitness aspirations. We need to be realistic and have a healthy attitude to food and working out, and our appearance generally, and try to surround ourselves with positive people in this respect if we are to maintain a healthy and positive outlook.

If you suspect you or someone you know has an eating disorder, then you should contact your GP. He or she will tell you where you can get help; many hospitals, for example, run specific clinics. You can also contact the Eating Disorders Association (www.edauk.com).

2 UNDERSTANDING YOUR BODY AND WORKING OUT

In my many years of experience as a personal trainer, it has given me real pleasure to see great results from clients who have previously exercised, but never had the results they hoped for. It would appear that many women want to train, but don't understand the mechanics behind the exercises or the energy systems used, for example, and this can significantly reduce the effectiveness of their workouts. A little knowledge can make a big difference, and so in this chapter I provide an overview of the body's main systems and their response to exercise. This information will help to contextualise the practical training information provided later.

The cardiovascular system, heart and lungs

Cardiovascular exercise (often referred to as aerobic exercise) involves moving the body by using its large muscles in a repeated manner. The cardiovascular system is the heart, lungs and circulatory system, and CV exercise will strengthen and condition the CV system. The heart is in fact a muscle, and will respond to training in the same way as any other muscle by becoming larger and stronger.

The two main measures of the heart's efficiency are stroke volume (the amount of blood the heart can pump around the body) and heart rate (the effort required to pump the blood).

Heart rate (HR) is measured in beats per minute (BPM), and your HR will decrease with regular CV training (*see* page 17 for HR intensities). Your maximum heart rate (HRMax) will be largely genetically determined, and calculating your HRMax (*see* page 53) will help you to train safely at the right intensity to achieve your goals. You cannot lower your HRMax.

MUSCLES AND CV TRAINING

It's important to realise that your heart, although the key determinant, is not solely responsible for improved CV fitness; this is because your oxygen transportation system, which includes your lungs, arteries, veins, capillaries and muscles, is an equally vital component.

Muscles, and in particular their constituent muscle fibres, will respond differently to the type of training they are subject to, with important consequences for body shaping and fitness efforts. After a sustained period of CV training, our bodies will adapt and produce, for example, more capillaries in our muscles. These can be seen as oxygen-carrying highways – the greater their mileage, the greater the quantity of oxygen that can be transported to our muscles to fuel improved CV efforts.

Energy systems

Our bodies are great machines and, like all machines, they need energy to power them.

We can generate energy via three 'energy systems'.

THE AEROBIC ENERGY SYSTEM

If you go for a steady-paced run you'll invariably be training aerobically. These workouts are often called 'steady state' because during them the body's energy demand is balanced by its energy supply, hence the steady state. Our hearts are able to pump sufficient oxygenated blood around our bodies to fuel our aerobic engines.

TOO MUCH AEROBIC TRAINING FOR THE 'CELERY' CAN LEAD TO A SHAPE-LESS PHYSIQUE

Body shapes that emphasise aerobic training may compromise any desired muscle gain efforts (see page 45). The main exceptions are the 'apples/pears' who wish to shed fat and reveal their muscles – in their case, a high level of aerobic exercise is recommended.

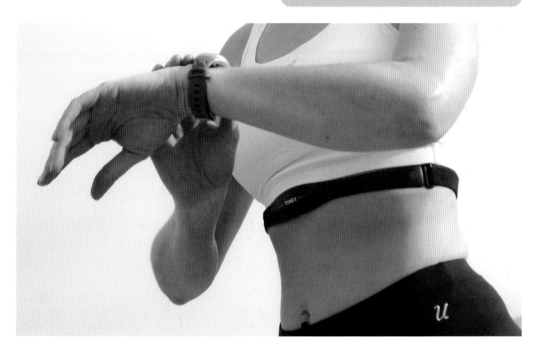

Aerobic energy is produced when oxygen combines with glycogen (carbohydrate), proteins and fats and is broken down by enzymes in our muscles to generate energy.

THE ANAEROBIC ENERGY SYSTEMS

If you've ever had to sprint after the bus, or you have tried to run up the stairs in the Underground, you will have already experienced anaerobic training! This type of energy can only be sustained for relatively short durations. There are two anaerobic energy systems: the immediate anaerobic system and the short-term anaerobic system.

The immediate anaerobic energy system

The immediate anaerobic system has no reliance on oxygen and supplies explosive energy, such as that required for a squat or golf swing. This energy lasts no more than 10 seconds. It relies on stored energy sources – for example, creatine phosphate – in our muscles and a chemical reaction to fire it up. Lifting a set of weights or sprinting 40m are examples of this energy system in action.

The short-term anaerobic system

This energy system produces high-powered (but not flat-out) energy for up to 90 seconds. It also relies on stored energy sources (body chemicals). However, as the one and a half minute mark nears, oxygen takes on an increasing role in attempting to keep the short-term anaerobic engine running. After 30 seconds, 20 per cent of the energy produced is done so aerobically, and after 60 seconds this is 30 per cent. As the 90-second mark nears, no amount of oxygen gulping will save our anaerobic engine and we will grind to a potentially painful out-of-breath halt. A tennis rally or a circuit training workout, or short burst of intense running, are examples of this energy system in action.

> ## Training tip
>
> It is important to realise that aerobic and anaerobic training targets different muscles fibres (see page 17–18) and in doing so can have a significant effect on the way our bodies 'shape' up.

Muscles and muscle fibre

There are more than 430 voluntary muscles and over 250 million muscle fibres in the body. Muscle fibres are bundles of cells, which are held together by collagen (connective tissue). Each fibre consists of a membrane, numerous nuclei and thousands of myofibrils (inner strands) that run the length of the fibre. In order

Table 3 Levels of CV exercise intensity and their effect on muscle fibre			
	Light (walking)	**Moderate (jogging)**	**Intense (running)**
Energy system	Aerobic	Aerobic	Aerobic/anaerobic
Energy source	Fat and carbohydrate	Carbohydrate and fat	Carbohydrate and fat
Heart rate (BPM)	<120	120–150	>150
Breathing	Easy	Can still talk	Difficult to talk
Muscle fibre recruited	Slow twitch – type 1	Type 1 and fast twitch – type IIa	All

to perform a sports skill or fitness activity, numerous muscles and muscle fibres interact. These are 'controlled' via electrical messages sent from the brain through the spinal cord and out to our muscles. When these signals reach the muscles, a chemical reaction occurs which results in muscular action. Depending on the physical activity and the chemical reaction, this muscular action can be short-lived, or longer-lasting (*see* energy systems on page 14).

There are three main types of muscle fibre, and these respond to training differently. This response will significantly affect how our body shape changes and how we adapt to fitness and sports training.

SLOW TWITCH TYPE I FIBRE

Type I fibres are designed to sustain relatively slow, but long-lived, muscular contractions. They are also known as slow twitch, slow oxidative (SO) or red fibres as they function for long periods on aerobic energy. They twitch at a rate of 10–30 per second.

FAST TWITCH TYPE II FIBRE

Fast twitch muscle fibres contract two to three times faster than slow twitch muscle fibres, producing 30–70 twitches per second. These fibres are also known as white fibres.

There are two basic types of fast twitch fibre:

- **Type IIa.** Type IIa or 'intermediate' fast twitch fibres are also termed 'fast oxidative glycotic' (FOG) because of their ability to display, when subject to the relevant training, a relatively high capacity to contract under conditions of aerobic or anaerobic energy production.
- **Type IIb.** Type IIb fibres act as 'turbo-chargers' in our muscles; they swing into action for high-power activity, such as a 40m sprint or heavy weight training. These fibres are also known as 'fast glycogenolytic' (FG) fibres. They rely almost exclusively on the immediate anaerobic energy system to fire them up. These are the fibres that any body type/shape wanting to increase muscle size should concentrate on (*see* page 82 for methods of training these fibres).

The endocrine system and its effects on body shape

You might not be aware of it, but training will have a significant hormonal effect on your body

> ### Training tip
>
> You should not be scared to lift heavy weights that target your fast twitch muscle fibres as these can build shapely muscles.

– working out will stimulate the production of these 'chemical messengers'. They are produced from a number of sites (endocrine glands) on the body – for example, the hypothalamus in the brain.

The major function of hormones is to change the rate of specific reactions in cells. Our muscles, like the rest of our bodies, are composed of cells and it is the way that certain hormones interact with these that is crucial to the way our bodies will adapt and shape up in response to training. The two key hormones in this respect are growth hormone and testosterone. They are termed 'androgens' and they serve an anabolic (stimulatory) function.

GROWTH HORMONE (GH) AND WORKING OUT

GH is released from the anterior pituitary gland in the brain soon after a workout starts. This hormone can be regarded as the 'fitness or sports hormone' because it is involved in numerous positive anabolic (growth) functions that will enhance the performance of our bodies. Specifically, GH contributes to bone, cartilage and muscle growth. This explains why it has been used as an illegal ergogenic aid in sport.

TESTOSTERONE AND WORKING OUT

Testosterone is primarily responsible for male sexual characteristics, but is also present in women in much smaller amounts. It's produced in the ovaries and adrenal glands. Testosterone interacts with GH to augment its release and also interacts with the nervous system. Because women have low levels of testosterone, they do not build muscle as easily as men. It is important to understand this relationship between gender differences and muscle growth, because many women avoid weight training as they fear the development of a muscular, bulky physique.

Women have on average 20 times less testosterone compared to men on a daily basis. Men produce 4–10mg a day.

- Both GH and testosterone levels of release are affected by the intensity of our workouts, and even the weight training system employed.

CORTISOL AND WORKING OUT

Cortisol is released from the adrenal glands; its levels are elevated by exercise. It stimulates protein breakdown, leading to the creation of energy in the form of glucose from the liver (*see* page 130 for more information on protein).

Metabolic rate and body shape

Your metabolic rate is essentially the amount of energy (calories) your body burns. This means the amount of calories your body needs to sustain itself for daily life – including work, rest and play. Exercise and the type of exercise you do can have a significant effect on metabolic rate and your body shaping efforts (*see* page 51).

There is a lot of debate about metabolism, and many women (and men) may blame a 'slow metabolism' for their weight gain. While this might not be the actual cause, women will more than likely have a slower metabolism due to their greater number of fat cells compared to men. Fat is 'lazy' body tissue and burns fewer calories than lean muscle tissue.

Metabolic rate comprises:

- Total Daily Energy Expenditure (TDEE): This refers to the totality of all the energy the body burns over a day.
- Resting Metabolic Rate (RMR): A very significant proportion (60–75 per cent) of TDEE is used to maintain RMR. RMR encompasses all those unseen and un-thought of essential bodily functions, such as heart, lung and

mental functioning. Calculations of RMR are made over a 24-hour period, but do not include the calories burned while sleeping.

- Thermic Effect of Feeding (TEF): The process of eating and digesting food generally burns around 8–10 per cent of TDEE, although this can be increased depending on the quantity and composition of food – TEF is higher after protein and carbohydrate intake, compared to fat.
- Activity: Physical activity can be the most variable component of TDEE, and has by far the most profound effect. Generally, physical activity accounts for around 15–30 per cent of TDEE and is regarded as a vital component of a weight loss programme.

Training tip

Physical activity is composed of general activity as well as formal exercise, and everyday activities such as taking the stairs instead of the lift, walking to the shops instead of driving, and losing the remote control, and even fidgeting, will all help to increase energy expenditure.

How to calculate your metabolic rate

Step 1 Calculate your RMR

Age:	18–30	31–60
	Multiply your weight in kg x 14.7 and add 496	Multiply your weight in kg x 8.7 and add 829
Example:	65kg individual 65 x 14.7 + 496 = 1451.5 RMR	65kg individual 65 x 8.7 + 829 = 1394.5 RMR

Step 2 Estimate your daily activity requirements in calories

Multiply your RMR by your daily activity level as indicated by one of the figures in the table below:

Activity level:	Defined as:	
Not much	Little or no physical activity	RMR x 1.4
Moderate	Some physical activity, perhaps at work 1 or the odd weekly gym visit	RMR x 1.7
Active	Regular physical activity at work and/or at the gym (three visits per week)	RMR x 2.0

Examples:
25-year-old weighs 65kg and has a moderate activity level – 1451.5 x 1.7 = 2466.7kcal
40-year-old weighs 80kg and has an active activity level – 1525 x 2.0 = 3050kcal

UNDERSTANDING ENERGY RELEASE FROM FOOD

We have looked at the body and energy systems, and now we need to look at how different foods can affect your health and body shape.

Kcal and calories

A kcal and a calorie supply the same amount of energy (that's why the terms can be used interchangeably). (Metric: 1 kcal = 1000 calories; Imperial: 1 calorie –1000c.)

Kilojoules

The kilojoule (kJ) is the international standard for energy; 1 kJ = 1000J.

A kJ is *not* the same as a kcal (or calorie) in terms of its energy provision. To facilitate your fat burning and dietary calculations and ease your understanding of food labels, you can convert kJ into kcal and vice versa using this calculation:

- To convert kJ into kcal divide by 4.2 – thus 200kJ = 48 cal (200/4.2).
- To convert kcal into kJ multiply by 4.2 – thus 100kcal = 420kJ (100 x 4.2).

> ## Training tip
>
> Forget faddy diets, and get-slim-quick gimmicks. In order to lose body weight, calories in (food eaten) needs to be lower than calories out. Creating a negative calorie balance is best achieved with workouts and dietary control.

Use the figures in Table 4 to gain an idea of how many calories you can burn during your workout. Exercises and other activity-based calorie burning can have a significant effect on weight loss (or weight gains). You'll need to factor in exercise expenditure figures when calculating your energy needs. See also post-exercise-induced calorie burning (*see* page 51); working out regularly can boost your daily calorie expenditure by as much as 20 per cent.

> ## Training tip
>
> There are 3500kcal in 0.45kg (1lb) of fat. Although this may sound an incredible number – when compared to the calories you burn in a workout – regular training can make a big difference.
>
> If you burned 300kcal a day through exercise and increased general activity, in a year you could theoretically remove 13.6kg of fat from your body.

Table 4 Energy costs of selected exercise methods

Activity	kcal/hour	Approx. kcal/min
Aerobics, high intensity	520	8.5
Cycling 16km/hour	384	6.4
Cycling 8.8km/hour	250	4.2
Rowing (moderate)	445	7.4
Swimming (fast)	615	10.2
Swimming for fitness	630	10.5
Weight training	270–450	4.5–7.5
Treadmill running (5.6min/km)	75	12.5
Treadmill running (3.8min/km)	1000	

The figures in Table 4 are based on a 65kg individual. If you weigh more, you'll burn more calories; if you weigh less, you'll burn fewer calories.

Women and ageing

Regardless of body shape we will experience decline in our physical function with age. Although this decline is particularly marked in sedentary women, it can be seriously challenged by the active. I have provided some reasons for physiological decline and their solutions.

1) DECLINE IN MUSCLE MASS AND MUSCLE FIBRE

We will all experience a 10 per cent decline in muscle mass between the ages of 25 and 50 and a further 45 per cent shrinkage as we reach our eighth decade if we do nothing about it. Decline in muscle tissue will lower our metabolic rate, thus increasing our chances of weight gain. Our strength and power will also be negatively affected, reducing our mobility.

Solution: Resistance train, and adjust diet accordingly (*see* pages 59 and 120).

2) LESS GROWTH HORMONE

One of the major consequences of a reduction in growth hormone production is a diminished level of protein synthesis. As protein is the key building block for muscle, this also leads to muscle shrinkage, with a consequent reduction in strength and power and shape.

Solution: As for point 1, plus (where appropriate) intense and consistent training.

3) DECLINE IN FAST TWITCH MUSCLE FIBRE

Fast twitch muscle fibre declines much faster with ageing than slow twitch fibre – by as much as 30 per cent between the ages of 20 and 80. This is because the nerves that control these fibres die off, with knock-on consequences for the fibres themselves. This will slow us down if we participate in speed-based sports and reduce the plumpness of our muscles.

Solution: As for points 1 and 2, plus some sports speed and power training.

4) REDUCED PRODUCTION OF CREATINE PHOSPHATE

Creatine phosphate is one of the premium ingredients for short-term physical activity. Production of this body chemical declines with age and, with less of it in our muscles, we will experience less energy for interval training and other stop-start activities such as tennis or squash.

Solution: Performing stop-start activities in training can maintain creatine phosphate levels, returning them to similar levels to those of the young.

5) REDUCED FLEXIBILITY

With age, soft tissue (muscles, ligaments and tendons) hardens and joints stiffen, increasing the potential for injury. This will affect our mobility and posture.

Solution: Regular stretching (*see* pages 32–5).

Training tip

It doesn't matter how old you are when you begin your exercise regime, your body will always respond and adapt to the training stimuli. Obviously, if you are in middle and older age and new to exercise (or retuning after a long break), you need to start slowly and build up exercise confidence and strength.

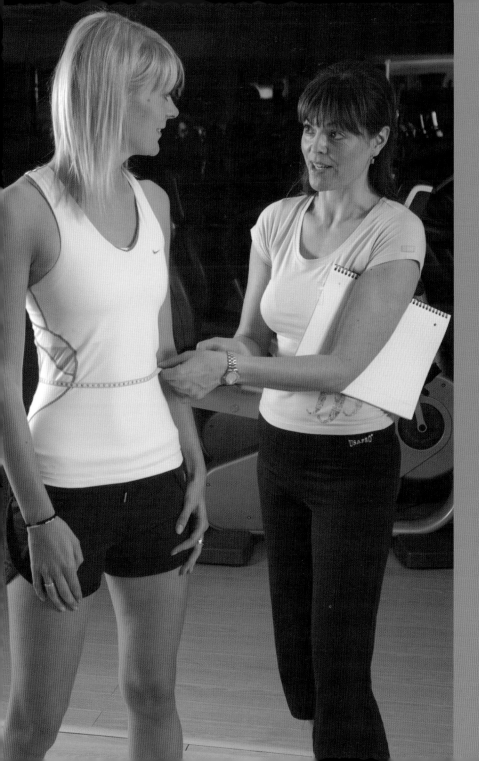

PART 2
TRAINING YOUR BODY SHAPE

3 WARMING UP AND COOLING DOWN

Now that you have identified your body type and your current body shape, I will show you how to go about training it. In this part of the book I'll tell you how to get the most from your exercise routine and which are the best exercises for your shape. I have divided it into warming up, pre-conditioning (that's training to train), CV, resistance training, other training and I have provided a comment on pregnancy and menopause. Where relevant, I have used the body shape symbols to help you identify the best exercises for you, but remember that how you shape up is also determined by your genes, your environment, your motivation and, crucially, your nutrition.

Women are generally more conscientious than guys when it comes to warming up and stretching. This is good as the warm-up is a crucial part of your workout. There has been a lot of controversy recently as to whether stretching before exercise has any real benefit – this is due to the fact that a held stretch has little direct relevance to the majority of more dynamic fitness and sports movements. The fitness industry now accepts that a good warm-up that raises your body temperature and includes movements similar to those you will perform in your workout is much more important for all modes of exercise. Stretching is best done at the end of your session (or in separate workouts) when muscles are warm (*see* page 32).

To warm up you should perform dynamic (but controlled) movements after you have raised your body temperature with 5 minutes of CV activity. These should prepare all the muscle groups that you will be working in the main part of your workout – for example, shoulder circles, marching on the spot, arm circles, calf raises and knee bends, and walking lunges. These exercises would be suitable for aerobics and step workouts – running and rowing, for example.

For weights workouts, although you may wish to incorporate some of these and other movements, the key will be to perform some reps (8–10) at a light weight prior to performing your designated sets, reps and weight on the exercise you are going to perform.

Suitable dynamic warm-up exercises for selected fitness activities

ROWING

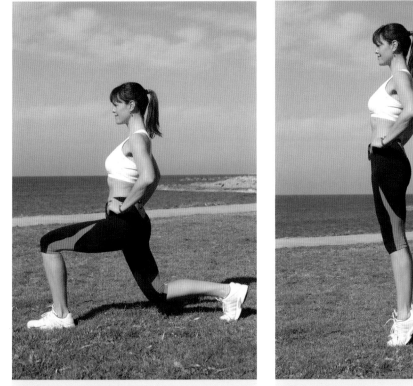

Fig. 3.1 *Lunges*

Fig. 3.2 *Calf raises*

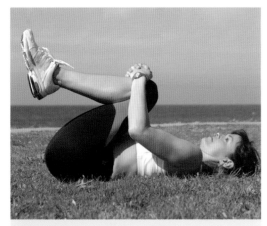

Fig. 3.3 *Lower back stretch*

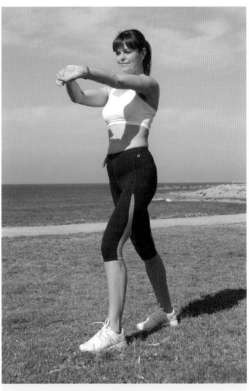

Fig. 3.4 *Forearm stretch*

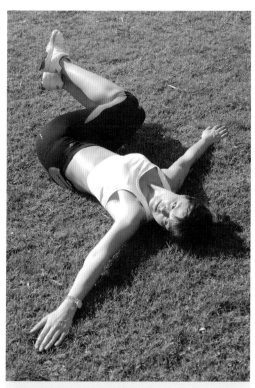

Fig. 3.5 *Lying side-to-side trunk rotations (to the right)*

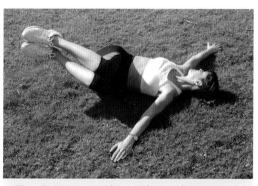

Fig. 3.6 *Lying side-to-side trunk rotations (to the left)*

RUNNING

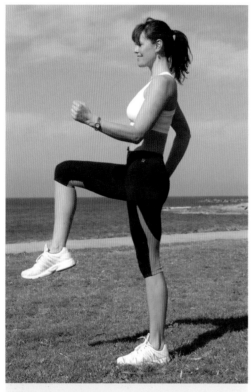

Fig. 3.7 *Marching on the spot*

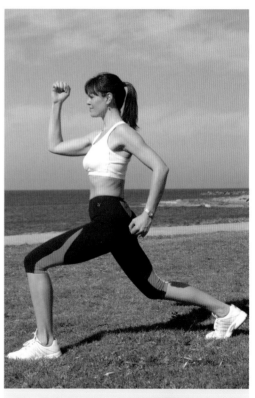

Fig. 3.8 *Simulated running action*

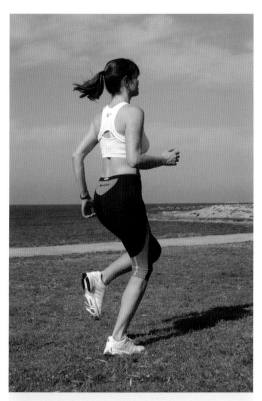

Fig. 3.9 *Backward running*

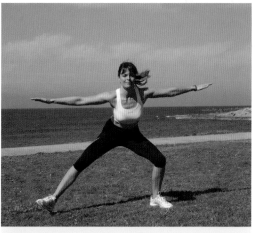

Fig. 3.10 *Sideways running*

WARMING UP FOR SPORT

The dynamic warm-up should include exercises similar to those identified for both rowing and running, plus those specific to the particular sport; for example, simulated racquet swings for tennis, lunges and sideways and backwards running, and throwing actions for netball.

For most activities, 5 minutes of low-intensity running should first be performed; this will turn on the myriad of physiological processes needed for an effective workout. With weight training, there is less need for CV preparation as noted.

The cool down

After CV, resistance and sports workouts you should cool down with some gentle CV activity, and perform some stretches to the muscles you have targeted.

Stretching

Although stretching before your workout is less important, it is still a vital part of your workout routine. It has many benefits: stretching after exercise or during a yoga or stretch class will reduce muscle tightness, aid recovery and reduce the risk of injury. Stretching also helps with the ageing process by keeping the physique lithe and supple.

If you are just starting out on a workout programme, then stretching is even more important. It would obviously be inadvisable for an out-of-condition, overweight 'apple' to begin her workout programme with a relatively high-intensity warm-up. In this case, time must be spent preparing her body for workouts, and stretching will serve a pre-conditioning value in this case.

As indicated, stretching slowly is less relevant than might be thought before a workout when more dynamic and specific preparation is better. However, stretching is still important after workouts, and to maintain flexibility and aid relaxation. Here is a very general post-exercise stretch sequence for all body shapes.

Range of movement

Whether you are training for fitness or sport, your muscles must be able to attain safely the positions (range of movement) required for their performance. Strengthening the relevant muscles is equally important (*see* pre-conditioning – page 37).

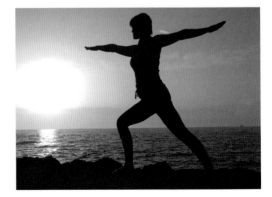

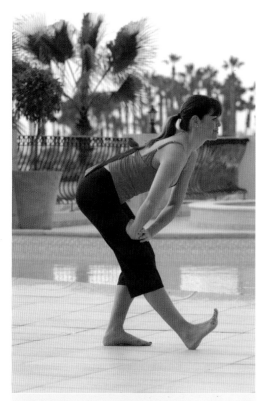

Fig. 3.11 *Hamstring stretch*

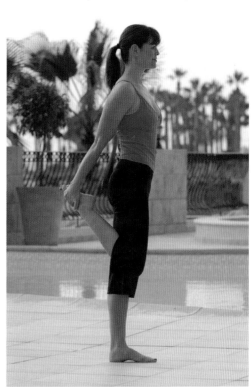

Fig. 3.12 *Quad stretching*

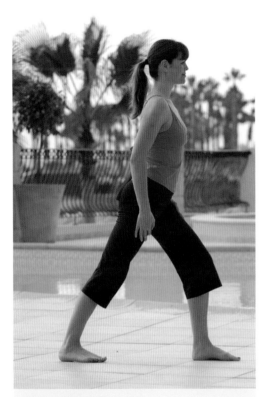

Fig. 3.13 *Calf stretch*

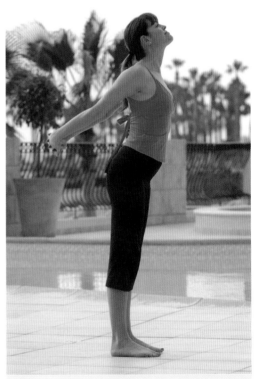

Fig. 3.14 *Chest stretch*

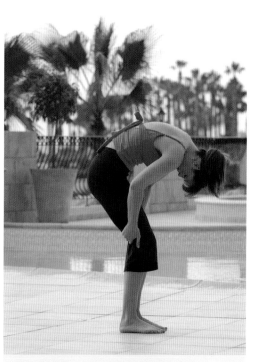

Fig. 3.16 *Lower back stretch*

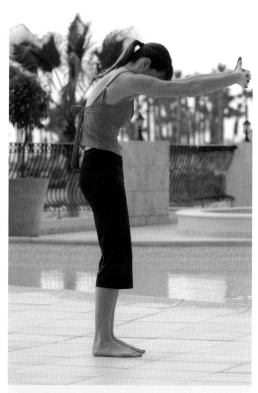

Fig. 3.15 *Upper back stretch*

Training tip

Hold the stretches for 20 seconds and gently ease into them. Keep warm while doing them and stop if you feel any sharp pains – although a little discomfort is to be expected.

Yoga and Pilates

Yoga and Pilates have really gained popularity with many sports professionals and celebrities, and they often name one or the other as an important part of their training. Both yoga and Pilates are excellent for developing body awareness. This is a crucial part of taking control of your fitness. Pilates focuses on core (abdominal and back) strength and stability, and so is a wonderful pre-conditioning (and, of course, conditioning) system. It uses bodyweight and flex bands for resistance, for example, and can become very challenging as you progress through the levels. Most of my female clients have loved the girdle effect that Pilates can have if performed correctly. This is perfect for an 'apple' needing to shrink her mid section, or an hourglass looking to emphasise her waist.

Yoga has many different forms, and has a strong emphasis on meditation and breathing. In this way it is a wonderful stress reliever, and can also have a strong toning effect on the body. Yoga, like Pilates, uses bodyweight for resistance, and you only have to look at a regular yogi's arms to see what effect it can have! Both Pilates and yoga are wonderful for stretching, toning and developing good levels of strength (*see* pages 85–95 and 96–101 for sample Pilates/yoga workouts.)

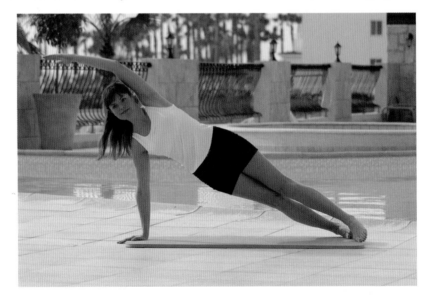

4 TRAINING TO AVOID INJURY (PRE-CONDITIONING)

You might never have heard of pre-conditioning or pre-training. You might think, 'Isn't going to the gym enough to train?' Well, it is in many ways, but in a number of others it isn't. Pre-conditioning comes from the sports training world, but its philosophy and practice are just as important for 'everyday' fitness training, whatever your body shape. Basically, pre-conditioning is the training you do to significantly reduce injury and 'deal with' any previous injuries. It runs consistently in the background to your workout programme and provides the foundation strength and resilience on which your body can build more substantial fitness.

Why pre-condition?

Here are some examples:

Celery
As a 'celery' you might have a light frame, a frame that is therefore potentially more prone to strain injuries. A relevant pre-conditioning programme involving resistance exercises could help prevent these, by strengthening your bones, muscles, ligaments and tendons.

Apple
As an 'apple', you may be overweight and equally prone to joint strain; therefore a pre-conditioning CV routine could prepare your body and prevent injury, by reducing weight. (Note: You would need to select the appropriate CV exercise equipment option and the right intensity programme – see page 53.)

Women's skeletal make-up does make us prone to certain injuries that could be brought on through an inappropriate exercise selection. Our wider hips and their effect on the knee joint is a specific case in point (see 'Q angle' below). Consequentially, we are more prone to anterior cruciate ligament (ACL) strain than men. The ACL is one of four ligaments that are critical to the stability of the knee joint. A ligament is made of tough fibrous material and functions to control excessive motion by limiting joint mobility. Without ligaments to control the knee, the joint would be unstable and prone to dislocation. One piece of American research indicated that female basketball players are four times more prone than males to ACL damage. To counteract this, women need to work on hamstring and quadriceps strength. Squats, however, may not be suitable for some women due to the stress they place on the knee joint and its ligaments. Other exercises, such as lunges or leg extensions and hamstring curls, could be better options. If in doubt, speak to a personal trainer or sports/weights coach.

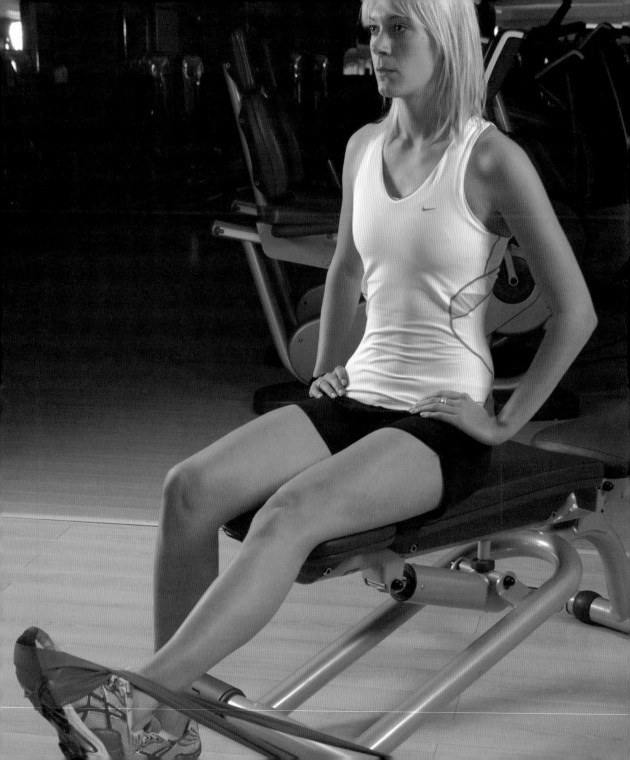

A note on female sports players

If you play club netball, you'll probably have seen many players suffer from knee and ankle problems. Many of these can be attributed to the way that women land from jumps. Female sports players should therefore be introduced more carefully than men to plyometric (jumping) training and sports for similar reasons to ACL damage, and because their hamstring muscles (which provide stability to the knee joint) are generally weaker than men's and need relevant strengthening. Preparing a woman's body to withstand plyometric training should involve suitable leg weights' exercises, such as hamstring curls, and involve a progressive programme of low-impact jumps to prepare them for more intense exercises. Suitable exercises would include jumps performed on the spot, such as jump squats, split jumps and straight leg jumps. Time must also be spent with your sports coach learning the correct jump technique.

What should you incorporate in your pre-conditioning programme?

it is impossible to provide an answer for everyone, but I'd recommend that you speak to a personal trainer, relevant sports coach or physio. Explain to them what training you are doing, and your training and injury history; from this, they should then be able to select appropriate exercises for you. They should of course reference your body type and current shape.

Posture

It is also relevant at this stage to point out that posture is very important when training. Many women tend to have inwardly rotated (round) shoulders due to stress, carrying and nursing children, and desk-bound office work. This posture could cause injury when, for example, lifting weights overhead.

To check your posture, turn sideways on to a mirror or ask a friend to photograph you

> ### Training tip
>
> The Q-angle is a measure of the angle between the quadriceps muscle on the front of the thigh and the patellar tendon at the knee. This angle is greater in a woman due to the fact that she has a wider pelvis than a man. This results in a naturally greater angle between the femur (thigh bone) and the tibia (shin bone), which predisposes the ACL to greater stress.

with your usual posture. There should be a straight line from your ear, to shoulder, to hip, to knee, to ankle. If your posture is poor, try Pilates exercises as part of your pre-training to re-balance (*see* page 85). You could also train in front of a mirror so you can check your alignment.

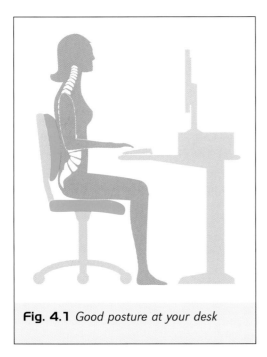

Fig. 4.1 *Good posture at your desk*

Training tip

Whatever your level of training, you must schedule rest periods into your workout routine. If you don't, you run the risk of injury and illness and compromised training gains. It is during recovery that your body adapts and grows stronger – not when you're training. This is why recovery and optimum nutrition are crucial – *see* page part 3.

An introduction to how to plan your work-outs is provided in chapter 9.

Selected pre-conditioning exercises related to body shape, fitness and selected sports activities

LEG EXTENSION (WEIGHTS) OR FLEX BAND

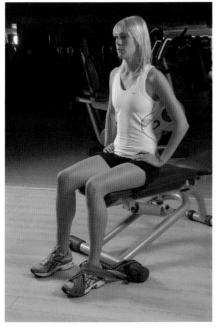

Method
Gradually increase the weight lifted to a medium to heavy weight, performing 2–4 sets of 6–10 repetitions with one minute's recovery between sets.

Pre-conditioning value
Stabilises and strengthens the knee joint.

Fitness and sports applicability
This exercise is for all.

Comments/tips related to body type/shape
- Suitable for independent left and right leg training for a more balanced strength development.
- Of use to all body types/shapes to reduce impact-related stresses on the knee.

(Note: Overweight women are best advised not to emphasise impact-based CV methods, such as running, in their training programmes in order to reduce potential joint stress.)

PILATES SHOULDER OPENERS

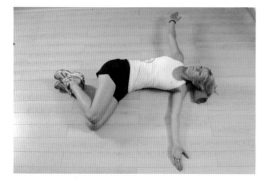

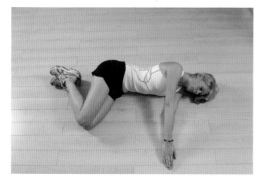

Method
Open and close three times, holding open for three breaths on final rep.

Pre-conditioning value
Improves shoulder stability and upper body posture.

Fitness and sports applicability
Great preparation for lifting weights and for correcting posture for all sports and fitness activities.

Comments/tips related to body type/shape
Can be included as a regular shoulder warm-up.

ECCENTRIC CALF RAISE

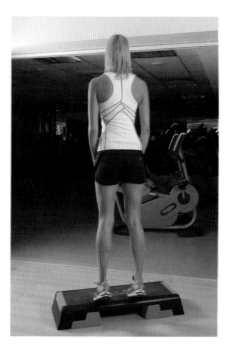 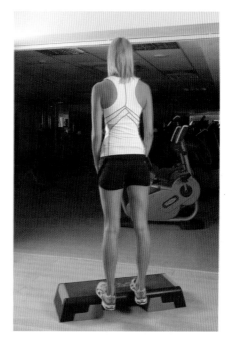

Method

This exercise emphasises the lowering phase of the movement. Lower to a slow 4 count. Gradually build up to a medium to heavy weight, performing 2–4 sets of 6–12 reps.

Pre-conditioning value

Strengthens Achilles tendons and calf muscles.

Fitness and sports applicability

Aerobics and dance, running and all running-based sports.

Comments/tips related to body type/shape

All body shapes could benefit from this exercise as Achilles problems are common among numerous sports and fitness trainers.

THE PLANK

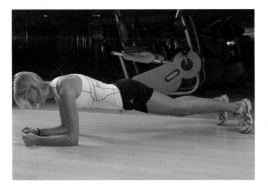

Method
Increase the length of the hold from 5 seconds to 60 and beyond as confidence and fitness improves. Do 2–6 reps.

Pre-conditioning value
Strengthens the core.

Fitness and sports applicability
All fitness and sports activities.

Comments/tips related to body type/shape
Back problems are common in both the fitness and sports worlds. The plank will develop core 'holding' strength, reducing the potential for injury when running or performing overhead weight lifting movements and those required for everyday life. The exercise is suitable for all body shapes.

TOP OF THE WORLD

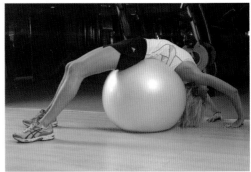

Method
Fit ball stretch – hold the stretch for 20 seconds and do 3 reps.

Pre-conditioning value
Stretches the whole body from tip to toe. Counteracts the pulling forward emphasis of desk work and driving.

Fitness and sports applicability
All fitness and sports activities.

Comments/tips related to body type/shape
Suitable for all body shapes.

Note: This exercise should be performed with a personal trainer for the first few times. Older people should take expert advice before performing.

5 CARDIOVASCULAR TRAINING

Most women wishing to lose weight will start with CV exercise, but often they train in the wrong 'zones' (*see* page 48) and have difficulty reaching their goals. As you will see in the resistance section, CV training is only a part of the bigger workout picture. It should form part of a balanced programme including weight training (and other exercise options).

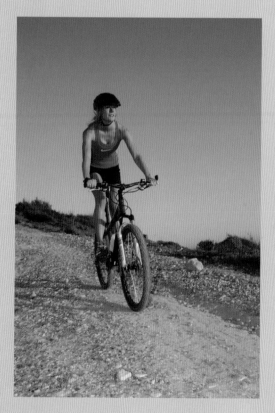

However CV exercise increases heart and lung function and can be a powerful calorie blaster. In this chapter I will show you how to get the very best out of your workouts.

Health benefits of CV exercise

CV training improves heart health. You might not realise it, but your heart is a muscle and it will respond to training in very much the same way as skeletal muscle by increasing in strength and size. With this growth it will be able to pump more oxygenated blood around your body (its stroke volume will be increased) with less effort (heart rate). Additionally, a healthy heart will make you less prone to a myriad of illnesses and diseases.

Body shapes and CV exercise

CELERY SHAPE
As a 'celery', your slim body and lighter frame make you very suited to CV exercise, particularly running, although pre-conditioning is still a must. Those of you looking to balance your body could consider swimming, as it is an excellent form of non-impact CV exercise that can add definition to the shoulders, giving you more shape. 'Celeries' who are already very slim or even underweight will need to bear in mind that CV exercise such as running

to build lean muscle tissue. The 'apples' among us need to take care to protect our (often delicate) ankles and knees, particularly if we are very overweight. For those heavier 'apples', rowing and cycling are a great place to begin CV training as body weight is supported, thus reducing impact. These two machines also use multiple muscles, creating potential for a high-calories burn. Swimming is another option that is perfect for all apple shapes and fitness levels.

CV exercise is crucial for 'apples' for heart health, and in order to reduce fat around the internal organs. For a beginner, walking is an excellent low to medium intensity form of exercise that can usually be tolerated well, even by overweight apple shapes (*see* page 53 for walking calorie-burn table). From experience, I highly recommend getting some new trainers to cushion your joints, and pre-conditioning the legs with calf raises and stretches whether walking or running. The lighter, fitter apple shape will have no problem adding running into her routine.

The fat burning fable

Forget the fat burning zone. Many women have read about, or heard of, the 'fat burning zone' (FBZ) and I often see women training in a leisurely fashion, without breaking a sweat, or even reading a magazine as they cruise along on the exercise bike! Unfortunately, their belief that slower, steady-paced exercise will give them a big fat burn is mistaken. The FBZ refers to relatively low-intensity CV workouts that last for more than 20 minutes. You might see reference to the 'zone' on posters in your local gym and hear about it from your personal trainer and gym instructor. Unfortunately, the concept of the FBZ is misleading and could result in you exercising ineffectively for optimum weight loss for your body shape.

The idea of a specific FBZ developed because 1) CV workouts carried out at a moderate intensity are both sustainable and achievable by those new to exercise, and 2) lower-intensity CV workouts seemingly burn more fat calories. You'll see from Table 5 that at low exercise intensities, 66.6 per cent of calories are derived from fat and 33.4 per cent from carbohydrate. Armed with this information, it's not too hard to see how low-intensity CV exercise as advocated by the FBZ can be championed as the best fat burner. However, in reality fat burning and attaining a negative/balanced energy balance (to lose or control weight) is best accomplished by training at higher CV intensities. This is because *total* calorie burn will be higher, and that is what really counts.

Interval training

Interval training is a fantastic way to improve your fitness levels, and can increase calorie burn

Table 5 Percentage calories burned between fat and carbohydrate

Exercise intensity	Percentage of kcal from:		Energy expenditure (kcal)	
	Carbohydrate	Fat	Per min	After 20 mins
Low	33.4	66.6	9.6	192
Medium	50.7	49.3	12.2	244
High	84	16	15	300
Very high	100	0	20.2	404

when compared to steady-paced CV workouts due to its higher intensity. This type of exercise can challenge your aerobic and anaerobic energy systems and will boost your fitness by, for example, making your heart and muscles more energy efficient at higher exercise intensities, which will make training at lower ones that much easier. Interval training is also useful for sport, as it can replicate certain activities – for example, a sudden sprint across the hockey field, or bursts of energy required to return a squash ball.

WHAT EXACTLY IS INTERVAL TRAINING?

Interval training divides periods of effort between periods of rest. You could, for example, complete 3 x 5-minute intervals on a rowing machine with 2 minutes' gentle rowing recovery between each interval. The speed at which you complete the intervals will be determined by your fitness level and training goals. Interval training is suitable for all body shapes, although a pre-conditioning phase and a base level of CV fitness must have been achieved first if performing high intensity anaerobic intervals. Table 6 gives a sample interval training workout.

This format can be adapted to cycling or rowing, for example. As your fitness progresses you can increase the speed, or lengthen the faster tempo interval – for example, from 2 minutes' jogging to 2 minutes 30 seconds. Or you can progress to 2 minutes' jogging and 2 minutes'

Table 6 Sample interval training workout suitable for beginners, involving running and walking

Duration	Treadmill pace	What it should feel like
5 mins warm-up	3–3.5 mph	Steady pace, gradually warming up the body, swinging the arms
2 mins	3.8–4.4 mph	Brisk but sustainable walking, able to hold a breathy conversation
2 mins	4.5–5 mph	Faster pace, OK to sustain for the 2 mins, but happy to go back to the recovery tempo
2 mins	3.8–4.4 mph	Recovery tempo – able to hold breathy conversation
2 mins	4.5–5 mph	Faster tempo – as before
2 mins	3.8–4.4 mph	Recovery – as before Can still talk
2 mins	4.5–5 mph	Faster tempo – as before
2 mins	3.8–4.4 mph	Recovery – as before
2 mins	4.5–5 mph	Faster tempo – as before
2 mins	3.8–4.4 mph	Recovery – as before
5 mins	3–3.5 mph	Cool down – breathing slows down to near start levels

walking, and so on. I have seen many people, who thought that they would never be able to run, start out with a similar programme, and progress to being regular (and fast) runners.

Burning calories with your feet up

You'll probably like the sound of this. But it only works if you CV train regularly three to four times a week, as doing this will result in a constantly elevated metabolic rate – by as much as 20 per cent. This is the result of what's known as excess post-exercise oxygen consumption (EPOC). I've touched on this a couple of times previously. Basically, when we perform a CV workout our body switches on and turns up numerous physiological processes, notably oxygen processing and consumption. Other related functions include the release of energy from muscle cells and specific hormones, such as GH and testosterone. These processes do not return to base line levels immediately after a workout; rather, they continue operating at a high level. Research identifies two EPOC phases: a very high one in terms of energy cost in the two hours immediately after our workout, and another of less intensity that lasts up to 48 hours. This all adds up to increased calorie burning, which will affect how your body shapes up.

Training tip

Importance of correct nutrition for CV training regardless of body shape

- Antioxidants (vitamins A, C, E and the minerals selenium and zinc, for example) can reduce the cellular damage created by CV work (see page 134 for more information on antioxidants), although recent research indicates that this may be less important among experienced CV exercisers.
- Water (for workouts lasting up to an hour) or sports (energy) drinks (for workouts longer than an hour) will optimise your CV training.
- Carbohydrate is needed to keep your muscle fuel (glycogen) stores stocked. Start this process immediately after your workout.
- Protein is needed to maintain muscle mass. If you only do CV, perhaps because you are training for a sports event such as a 5km run, then you should go for 1.4–1.6g a day per kg of body weight.

Detailed nutritional advice and strategies as they relate to body shape are provided in Part 3.

Intensity matters

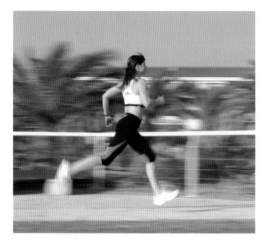

The intensity of exercise will have a profound effect on EPOC, with higher intensities creating a greater and more prolonged 'after burn'. This is one of the many benefits of interval training – your higher exercise intensity will turn up your EPOC. It has also been shown that splitting your training into multiple sessions in a day – for example, 20 minutes in the morning and 20 minutes in the evening, instead of one 40-minute session – increases overall EPOC.

All body shapes will turn up their metabolic rate with regular CV training (and resistance training – see page 59), which will benefit any desired weight loss goals. You will need to factor this in when calculating your 'energy balance' – for weight loss or lean weight gain.

Training tip

The higher your exercise intensity, the greater the potential for body shaping adaptation, everything else being equal – this is a consequence of the boost that your metabolism and endocrine system will get.

Note that, regardless of body shape, the use of very high-intensity sessions should be moderated in your training plans. Those new to exercise should obviously build their fitness up over a matter of months before tackling them. Nor, if you are an advanced trainer, should you think that training hard all the time is the best strategy – your body will eventually resent this and will fail to adapt as effectively as it would if you scheduled in easy and medium-intensity workouts, rest days and longer rest periods. You also risk injury if you over-train.

The importance of rest is covered in more detail in Part 3.

Training tip

If you are an overweight 'apple' or 'pear' and/or older, walking is a great way to boost your CV fitness. Take a look at the figures in Table 7.

Table 7 Calorie burning and walking

Walking speed	100lb female (45kg)	150lb female (68kg)	200lb female (90kg)
2mph 3.2km/hr	160 cal	240 cal	312 cal
3mph 4.8km/hr	210 cal	320 cal	416 cal
4.5mph 7.2km/hr	295 cal	440 cal	572 cal

Training intensities

I briefly referred to training intensity above. It is important to understand this concept, as it will help you maximise your calorie burn and fitness potential. Here we look at how to calculate your heart rate and your training intensity to help you maximise results from your exercise.

Calculative methods for establishing heart rate maximum and training zones

You'll probably be aware of the '220-your age' method of calculating your maximum heart rate (HRMax). You might also know that this formula can be inaccurate, by 10–15 per cent. This is because HRMax can be affected by stress, heat, hydration, fitness, motivation and even type of CV exercise – readings will invariably be higher on a rowing machine or treadmill and lower on a step machine or cycle due to the greater amount of muscle involved in generating energy on the former kit. Recently, a new calculative formula has been recommended as being much more accurate than the '220–your age'[i] one. For ease of use, this uses the following calculation: 207–(0.7 x your age). Using this formula, the predicted HRMax for a 30-year-old would be 186

[i] Med Sci Sports Exerc, 2007, May; 39(5): 822–9.

(this would compare with 190 using the 220–your age formula).

WHY DO YOU NEED TO KNOW YOUR HRMAX?

Knowing your HRMax calculated or actual enables you to train within designated heart rate zones (HRZ), knowing that your body is specifically responding. Knowing how hard your heart is working can significantly influence how your body shapes up and how motivated you are to maintain a workout programme.

Your heart rate will increase (in beats per minute) the harder you exercise. However, the fitter you are the more efficient (and stronger) your heart will be. This will mean that you'll be putting in less effort to complete your CV workouts, everything being equal. This is why it is important to know what HRZ you are in and what effect it is having on your body. This will leave you safe in the knowledge that you

are developing a certain type of CV fitness practically and systematically. To this end it is a good idea to purchase a heart rate monitor, but you will also find many pieces of gym equipment now have built-in heart rate monitors.

Only advanced CV trainers should perform a HRMax test – this requires incremental increases in exercise intensity, usually over 2-minute periods, until exhaustion is reached. At this point HRMax is achieved and measured in BPM.

Heart rate monitors

There are many heart rate monitors on the market nowadays, with some offering, for example, satellite tracking and distance covered. However, for the purpose of fitness training and monitoring, the simplest basic model will serve your needs. You may, however, wish to buy a monitor that allows you to download and track your progress.

Rate of perceived exertion (RPE)

If you do not have a heart rate monitor, then using the RPE system can also allow you to monitor your workouts. I have provided approximate heart rates for the levels (1–10) and describe 'how you should feel' at each level. It will take time for those new to it to develop consistent self-evaluation using RPE.

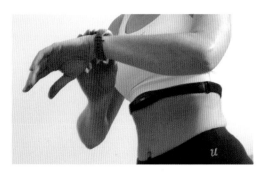

Table 8 Heart rate training zones	
Heart rate %HRMax	**Heart rate training zone and description**
50–60	'Light to moderate' – for the older and untrained. Low-calorie-burning potential. Primarily works slow twitch muscle fibre. Energy created exclusively aerobically.
60–70	'Everyday fitness zone' – this zone enables relatively comfortable and sustained CV exercise to be completed. It is often associated with the misleading belief that it is the best for fat burning – the reasons why this is *not* the case are explained on page 48. This zone also largely targets slow twitch muscle fibre. Also used as a recovery zone for those with advanced levels of CV fitness. It has a moderate- to high-calorie-burning potential. Energy is created virtually exclusively aerobically.
70–85	'Quality aerobic training zone' – this is the zone for intermediate and advanced trainers. It offers optimum calorie-burning potential for fat loss and great CV fitness development. Although the zone predominantly targets slow twitch muscle fibre, towards its upper end, with increased energy expenditure, it also involves fast twitch fibre, particularly IIa. These fibres will adapt and contribute towards generating increased CV power. This zone marks the transition into anaerobic training territory and can have a potentially significant post-exercise calorie-burning effect.
85–100	'High intensity training zone' – this zone is for advanced trainers and competitive athletes. It's not possible to exercise for long in it. All muscle fibre types are involved. It can burn proportionally high numbers of calories for its short duration, although this is largely attributable to its effect on elevating post-exercise metabolic rate. The upper end of this training zone really emphasises anaerobic energy production and targets fast twitch muscle fibres.

Table 9 Rate of perceived exertion (RPE)		
Rating	**How does it feel?**	**Approx. % heart rate**
1	Rest	
2	Very easy	
3	Moderate, can comfortably talk	
4	More purposeful walking, able to chat but breathing faster	
5	Starting to become warm, able to hold a breathy conversation	50
6	Challenging, sustainable for at least 20 mins, able to hold sporadic conversation	60
7	Very challenging. Unable to hold a conversation but can answer questions in between breaths – you get much warmer and begin to sweat	70
8	Very tough, as if running for the bus, only able to use one-word answers. You get hotter and sweat more	80
9	Maximum effort – your breathing is hard and quick and you sweat heavily	90
10	Heart rate is very strong as it reaches maximum output. You can't talk and you need to stop	Maximum

Table 10 Sample CV programmes for fat loss

Note: The workout ideas in Table 10 assume that you are suitably pre-conditioned and have prior levels of fitness required to perform the workouts suggested.

Body shape	Training level	Suggested CV workout
	Beginner or overweight	(1) 40-min walk 60–70% HRMax RPE 6 (2) 30-min cycle 60–70% HRMax RPE 6 (3) 30-min swim 60–70% HRMax RPE 6
	Beginner or overweight	(1) 20-min row 60–70% HRMax RPE 6–7 (2) 30-min cycle 60–70% HRMax RPE 6–7 (3) 40-min fast walk 60–70% HRMax RPE 6–7
	Intermediate (have been CV training 2–3 times per week for at least 6 months)	(1) 45-min row/X trainer 65–75% HRMax RPE 7 (2) 40-min cycle with hills 65–75% HRMax RPE 7 (3) 40-min hill walk 65–75% HRMax RPE 7 (use treadmill for gradient) or 50-min fast walk outdoors
	Intermediate	(1) 40-min run or 2 x 20-min intervals (walk for 5 mins between the intervals) 70–80% HRMax RPE 7–8 (2) CV mix workout: 10-min run, 10-min cycle, 10-min row (straight from one machine to the next) 70–80% HRMax RPE 7–8 (3) 30-min run/walk interval session (*see* page 50 for sample session)

Table 10 Sample CV programmes for fat loss (cont.)		
Body shape	**Training level**	**Suggested CV workout**
	Intermediate–advanced (have been consistently CV training for at least 12 months)	(1) 60-min steady pace run 75–80% HRMax RPE 7–8 (2) 30-min interval training speed session, work at RPE 8–9, recovery at RPE 6 (intervals 7 mins, recovery 3 mins) (3) 50-min gym CV mix: X trainer, treadmill on incline, exercise bike, rower: 75–85% HRMax/RPE 8 Go straight from one machine to the next

Where a hill programme is noted you should try to keep the same heart rate/RPE during the climbs as you would on the flat. If cycling this could mean dropping down through the gears to lighten the pedal load and also slowing your cycling speed (RPM).

Always warm up and cool down after your workout and drink water throughout your sessions to ensure optimum hydration.

All body shapes aiming for fat loss should aim for a *minimum* of three CV sessions per week. Try to vary your CV work and mix up the modes.

6 RESISTANCE TRAINING

Many women mistakenly believe weight training or resistance training is mainly for men. They may skip weights altogether, or only lift very light weights for fear of 'bulking up'. One of my main aims with this book is to encourage women to learn to love resistance training since it is a powerful weapon in the fight against ageing and flab!

Weight lifting is not the only way to overload muscles to increase their strength, and shape. Hill running, body weight moves, yoga and Pilates, and certain exercise classes such as those involving weights moves to music (*see* page 104), are all forms of resistance training. With such a variety of options, you should be able to discover one or a combination of methods that suits your training goals, your body shape and your level of fitness.

When starting an exercise programme regardless of your body shape, it is crucial that you progress slowly and learn correct technique. In the gym, I would always opt for free weights (dumbbells or barbells) over resistance machines, as they are much closer to everyday life – for example, carrying heavy shopping bags, or lifting a child from a car seat. Beginners should take care when selecting the weight to lift to prevent injury and should start out with very light weights so that the body can adjust slowly to the routine. Always use slow, controlled moves when learning new techniques, and don't be afraid to ask a trainer for advice.

Selecting the 'right' weights exercises

There are literally thousands of weights and resistance training exercises to choose from. Some work large muscle groups, such as the squat and the bench press (compound or multi-joint exercises), while others target smaller muscles such as the biceps curl (isolation or single-joint exercises). The exercises you select and the weight training system you use will have a significant effect on how your body responds to your workouts (*see* also training systems and hormonal response to weight training, pages 14–23).

COMPOUND EXERCISES

Compound exercises work more than one large muscle group, across a number of joints – for example, the squat, lunge or chest press. These exercises are more intense, and require more energy (effort) than isolation exercises such as a bicep curl (which target one muscle). Compound exercises are a great time-efficient challenge for all body shapes. These should become your 'staple diet' of weight lifting exercises.

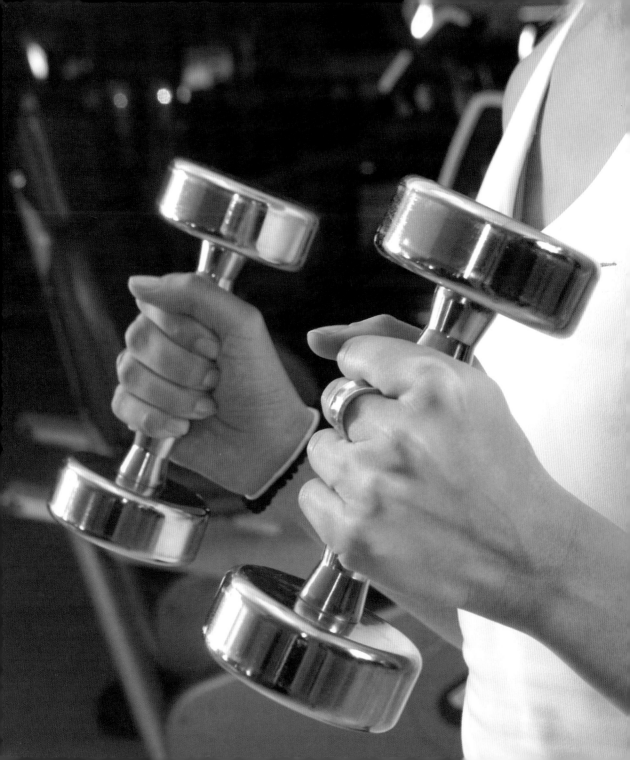

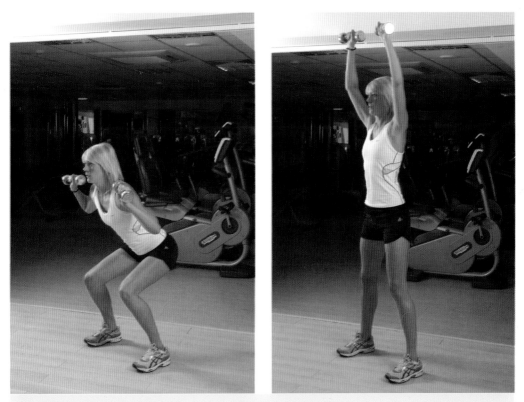

Fig. 6.1 *Squat with shoulder press (compound exercise)*

ISOLATION EXERCISES

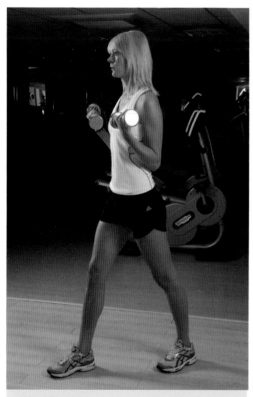

Fig. 6.2 *Bicep curl*

Isolation exercises, such as the biceps curl, are best left to the end of your workout if you perform them, as they do not require as much energy to complete as compound exercises.

Overweight 'apple' and 'pear' figures will benefit more from compound exercises, due to the exercise's increased energy requirements, and a slim 'celery' or un-toned 'hourglass' will appreciate the potential to help build shape and definition. It should be noted, however, that isolation exercises can be crucial for pre-conditioning purposes and avoiding injury (*see* page 37–44) for all body shapes.

> ## Training tip
>
> Muscles are active tissue and require energy all day long. Muscle is a calorie burner – for every 0.45kg increase in lean muscle mass, you could burn an additional 30 calories a day.

Knowing what to lift

Many women are unsure of what weight to lift, and generally will tend to go for weights that are too light due to the fear of bulking up. Don't worry, this will not happen – unless you are training very specifically, diet accordingly and have the 'right' genetics. The following guidelines will give you a good idea as to what's a heavy, medium and light weight. This is important because the amount of weight you lift, plus the number of sets and repetitions, will have a significant effect on how your body adapts to the stimulus.

I have indicated the intensity of the weights as a percentage of one repetition maximum (1RM) – the maximum you could lift once on any one exercise. Those new to weight training should not attempt to find their 1RMs.

- Light weight (LW) – less than 65 per cent 1RM – approximates to a weight you could lift 10–15 times before fatigue sets in.
- Medium weight (MW) – 65–75 per cent 1RM – approximates to a weight you could lift 7–10 times before fatigue sets in.
- Medium heavy/heavy weight (MH/HW) – 75–85 per cent 1RM – approximates to a weight you could lift 5–7 times before fatigue sets in.
- Heavy weight (HW) – 85–100 per cent 1RM – approximates to a weight you could lift less than 5 times.

(Note: These are approximations – the number of repetitions you are able to perform will be governed by your current level of strength and fitness.)

Muscular action and strength development

It can be all too easy to complete a weights workout and not fully understand the effects it will have on our bodies. We might be bliss-fully unaware of the different types of muscular actions we can use to develop tone, shape and strength. I've identified these as 'strength types' below. They are suitable for all body types and shapes, as long as the individual is pre-conditioned, has mastered exercise technique, and is at the right stage in their training.

- Isotonic muscular action. Isotonic muscular action involves movement and incorporates 'concentric' and 'eccentric' actions. Curling and lowering a dumbbell when performing a biceps curl and running are examples of isotonic muscular actions.
- Concentric muscular action. A concentric contraction occurs when a muscle shortens as it contracts to create movement. It's the most common direction of effort for resistance and CV exercise. During a biceps curl, the biceps contract concentrically to lift the weight.
- Eccentric muscular action. An eccentric muscular action involves the lengthening of a muscle as it contracts to create movement. During a biceps curl, the biceps extend eccentrically to lower the weight.

Isometric muscular action

During an isometric exercise no movement occurs. This is the result of opposing muscle groups working against each other, such as the biceps and triceps. Clasping your hands in front of your chest and pressing them together is an example of an isometric contraction. This type of training is not widely practised, as it is

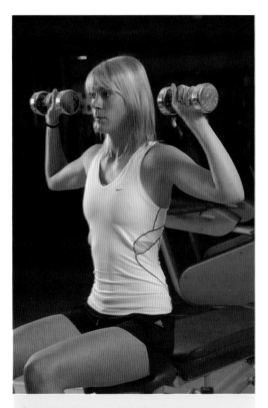

Fig. 6.3 *During the seated dumbbell shoulder press the core muscles work isometrically to hold the trunk in position*

difficult to measure its overall effect on muscle strength. However, isometric muscle actions are involved in some way in nearly all everyday, fitness and sports activities. For example, when performing a seated dumbbell shoulder press, the muscles of the core (abdominal and back muscles) work isometrically to hold the trunk in position.

Isokinetic muscular action

Isokinetic muscular action involves moving a pre-set resistance (concentrically and/or

Training tip

Resistance training targets your nervous system as well as your muscles. In fact, it's estimated that as much as 20 per cent of the 'strength' required to perform a common weight training move, like the bench press, results from nervous activity. In time, an exercise becomes so 'patterned' into the brain (and consequentially the muscles) that less effort is required to complete it. This will slow training progression as the neuromuscular system puts in less effort to do the job. This is why you must constantly change, progress, adapt and cycle your training.

eccentrically) over a full or part range of movement. Isokinetic resistance training machines exist in some gyms, although the majority of fixed weight installations are isotonic. Isokinetic machines are often used for injury rehabilitation purposes.

By varying the type of muscular action involved you can continually stimulate your muscles (and mind), which will bring about optimum adaptation and will also avoid training stagnation.

Training tip

The power of suggestion
Tell yourself that you are getting stronger and that your training is working to change your body shape or make you a better sports player. Research indicates that those with a positive training outlook and belief in what they are doing will get greater results than those who don't.

Keep changing your routines to get the most from your weight training

Many women discover exercises that they enjoy, and which may have given them great results, and so they continue doing them – believing they will get more of a good thing!

Unfortunately, this is not quite so, because as the body adapts to an exercise, less mental and physical stimulation is required to perform it, and so the benefit is greatly reduced. To prevent this stagnation, change your workout every 6 to 8 weeks. This change could be made by upping the weight, or changing your body position. For example, performing the chest press on a bench, and then changing to an exercise ball. Or squatting without weights, and then adding dumbbells. Perhaps static lunges and then walking lunges, or bicep curls, and then hammer curls (palms face in). This also applies to the number of sets and reps you use and the weight training system. If you are a beginner, you will start with single sets, and progress to 2 and then 3 sets of each exercise.

What equipment will I need?

The beauty of the resistance exercises I have provided is that they can be adapted for home or gym use. If you are training at home, some adjustable dumbbells (not a can of beans!) or a flex band, and an exercise ball (also called a Fit ball or Swiss ball) are all you will need. And many of the exercises require nothing but your body weight. However, I do recommend using weights in addition to ensure you get the best results.

Training your body shape – the resistance exercises

I have selected the most effective resistance exercises, all of which can be done at home or in the gym, with minimum equipment. On page 82 you will find sample workouts using a variety of these exercises for your body shape.

TRICEP BENCH DIPS

Targets

The back of the arms (triceps) and the shoulders (deltoids).

Method

- Stand with your back to a bench or sofa, with your feet a stride's length in front of it, and your hands on the edge supporting your body weight (palms down, thumbs inwards).
- Inhale. Bend your arms to slowly lower your bottom towards the floor until your upper arm is parallel to the floor.
- Exhale to push your body back up to the start position.

Training tips

Keep your neck long and eyes forward. As you progress, you can keep the legs straight throughout for extra resistance.

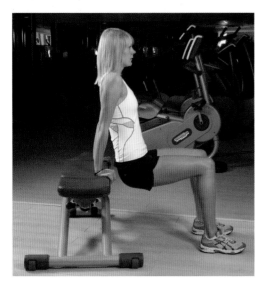
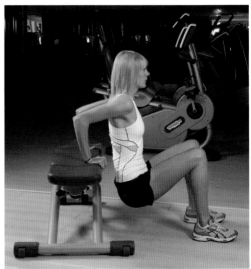

SQUAT WITH SHOULDER PRESS

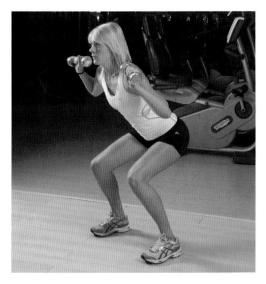

(Note: These can be performed separately.)

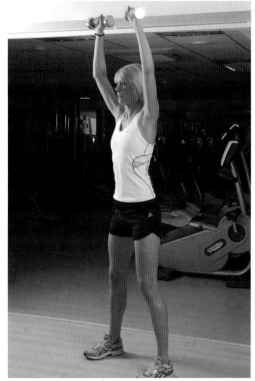

Targets
The legs and bottom, plus the shoulders.

Method
- Stand with feet hip to shoulder-width apart, bend your elbows to bring weights up to shoulders, palms forward.
- Inhale to bend knees, taking hips towards the floor.
- Exhale and push body back up, as you begin pressing dumbbells overhead until arms are almost straight.
- Return weights to shoulders and begin second squat.

Training tips
Keep knees in line with second toes, be careful not to let your knees roll in. It may be worth asking a trainer to check your technique. Keep abdominals drawn in throughout, and be careful not to arch your back.

THE PRESS UP

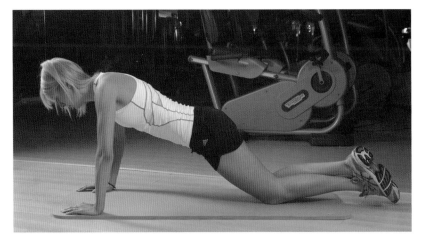

Targets
The chest muscles and the triceps.

Method
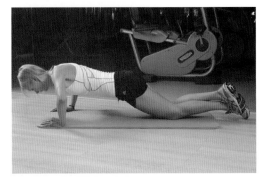

- Place hands under shoulders, and legs out straight with weight on your toes. If this is too challenging, bend knees as shown in the illustration.
- Keep your back straight, and inhale to lower chest towards the floor, bending your elbows.
- Exhale to press back up to start position.

Training tips
Keep abdominals tight throughout, and try to keep back straight and bottom tight. Placing hands wider apart works the chest more, and hands being narrower works the triceps more.

THE WALKING LUNGE

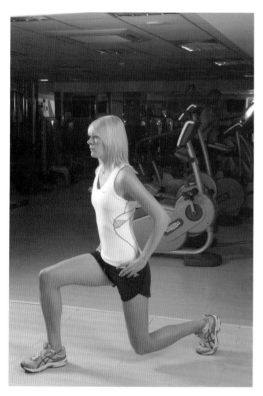

Targets

All leg muscles and also the core muscles (abdominals and back).

Method

- Stand tall, feet hip-width apart with navel drawn in.
- Take a large step forwards and bend knees until front thigh is parallel to the floor. Hold for 1 second.
- Raise your body up to return to starting position, lifting your back leg forwards to repeat the lunge with this leg.
- Continue lunging forward, alternating between legs.

Training tips

Keep abdominals engaged, and ensure your front knee stays in line with second toe of the front foot. Dumbbells can be held at arms' length for added resistance.

EXERCISE BALL CHEST PRESS

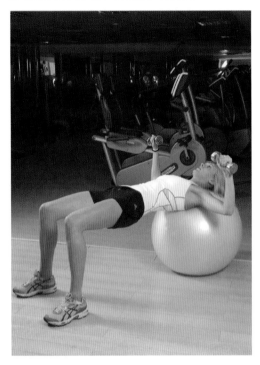 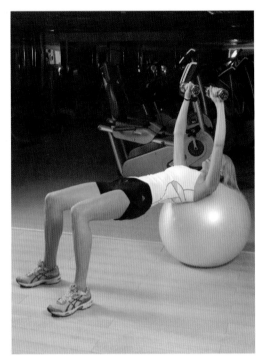

Targets
Front of the chest and triceps. Using the ball works the bottom and core muscles to a greater extent.

Method
- Lie with your shoulders and head supported on the ball, feet hip-width apart and buttocks engaged to keep hips up.
- Keeping palms facing forward, lower dumb bells out until elbow is at shoulder height, at a right angle.
- Exhale to press weights upward until hands are above shoulders.
- Inhale to control back down to start position.

Training tips
Ensure you keep squeezing the buttocks throughout, as this gives good alignment, and also tones your bottom at the same time.

BACK EXTENSION

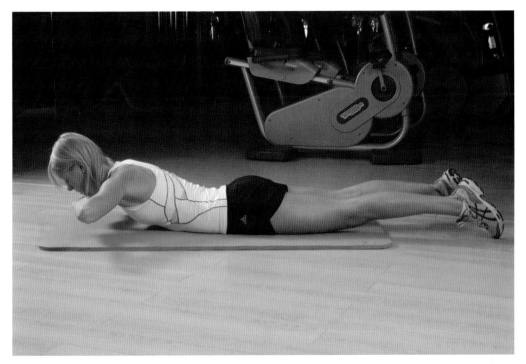

Targets

All back muscles.

Method

- Lie on your stomach with your hands palms down, fingers touching, under your chin.
- Exhale and raise head, shoulders and hands off the floor.
- Inhale to return to start position.

Training tip

Draw abdominals in as you lift, and use slow, controlled movement.

SIDE LUNGE WITH WOOD CHOP

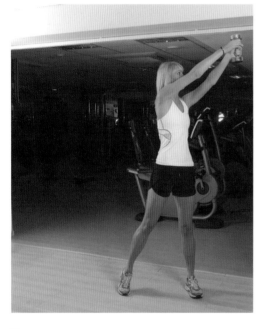 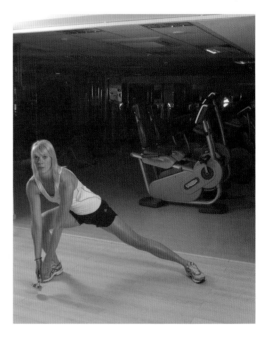

Targets
The inner thigh, leg and waist muscles.

Method
- Stand with feet shoulder-width apart, holding a weight (a 5kg medicine ball is ideal) in both hands, up above your left shoulder, as if holding an axe in preparation to chop some wood.
- Step out to the right and bend your right leg into a half squat, as you simultaneously swing your weight (axe) diagonally down past your right knee.
- Rise up to the start position and repeat in both directions.

Training tips
Beginners start with no weight, and progress. Stop briefly at beginning and end position rather than swinging back and forth. Keep abs tight throughout.

PLIE SQUAT WITH LATERAL RAISE

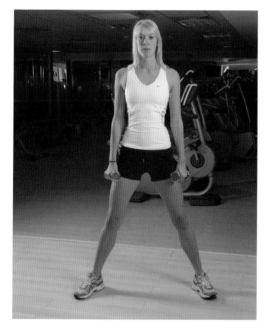 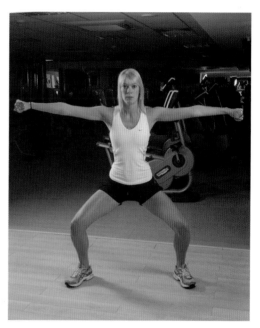

Targets

The bottom, inner/outer thigh and shoulder muscles. (Note: These two exercises can be performed individually as well.)

Method

- Stand with feet wide, toes turned out, holding dumbbells by your side, palms inwards.
- Tighten your buttocks and abdominals as you bend your knees out to the side, while simultaneously lifting your arms out to the sides to shoulder height.

- Straighten legs to return to start position as you control the weights back down by your side.
- Exhale arms up, inhale down.

Training tips

Keep buttocks squeezed throughout, and keep back straight while maintaining its natural curves. To progress add an extra rep (no arms) and hold at bottom position then squeeze bottom to 'pulse' halfway up and down 15 times.

EXERCISE BALL GLUTE RAISE

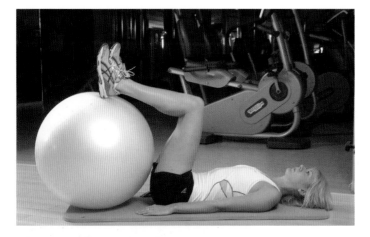

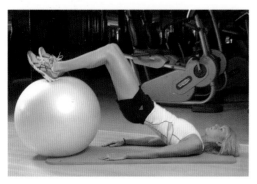

Targets
The bottom and the back of the thighs.

Method
- Lie on your back with your feet on top of an exercise ball (or bench), keeping your hands down by your sides.
- Exhale to squeeze bottom, lifting hips up until body is in a straight line.
- Inhale to lower halfway back down and continue smoothly on to next lift.

Training tip
Squeeze your bottom, abdominals and pelvic floor as you lift, and try to keep the ball as still as possible. A bench or chair is fine if you do not have a ball to hand.

BICEPS CURL

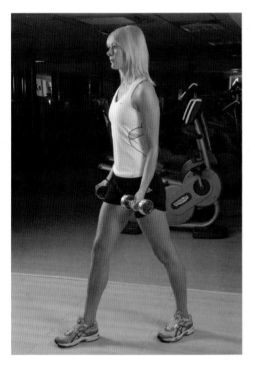 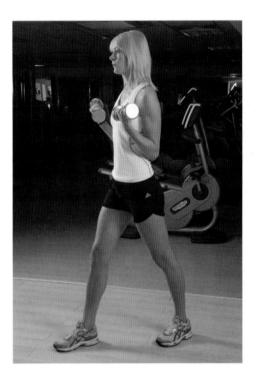

Targets
The muscles on the front of the arm (the biceps).

Method
- Stand with one foot forward, feet hip-width apart, and dumbbells held by your sides.
- Exhale and bend elbows, bringing dumbbells close to shoulder level. Do not turn the wrists in – maintain natural alignment.

- Inhale and slowly lower dumbbell back to start position.

Training tips
Try to keep your torso still and do not rock back and forth. Keep abdominals drawn in throughout. Try turning palms/dumbbells in towards each other for variety, this 'hammer curl' slightly alters the emphasis on the biceps muscles.

REVERSE LUNGE

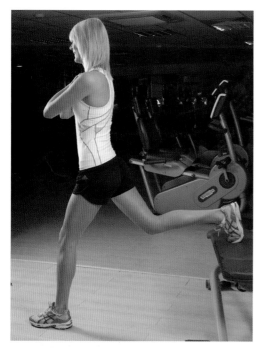 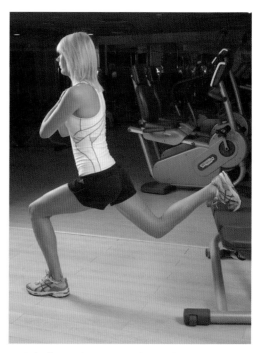

Targets
The bottom and thigh muscles.

Method
- Stand a stride's length in front of a chair or bench, feet hip-width apart.
- Place right foot on top of the bench, cross arms in front of chest.
- Inhale: bend your knees to lower hips towards the floor.
- Exhale and use your buttocks to drive you back to start position.
- Repeat on both legs.

Training tips
Keep chest lifted and abdominals drawn in throughout. Ensure your knee stays over your ankle and in line with second toe as it bends forward. Dumbbells can be held by your sides for progression.

UPRIGHT ROW

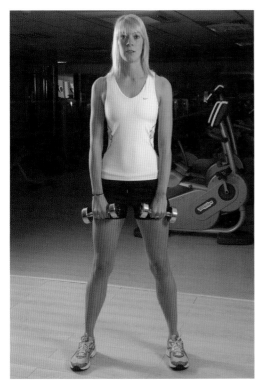
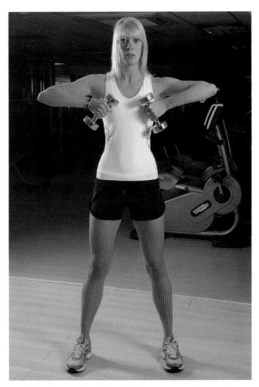

Targets

The shoulders and biceps muscles.

Method

- Stand with feet hip-width apart, legs softly bent, and dumbbells in front of thighs, palms facing in.

- Exhale and pull weights upwards to chest height, leading with the elbows.
- Inhale to slowly lower back to start position.

Training tips

This exercise can easily be performed at home with a resistance band or tube as an alternative to dumbbells. Try to keep your wrists in alignment with your forearms.

REVERSE FLYE

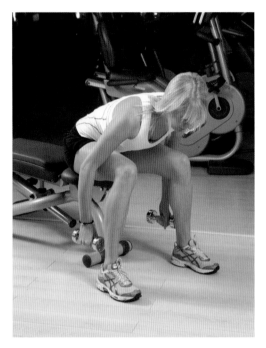 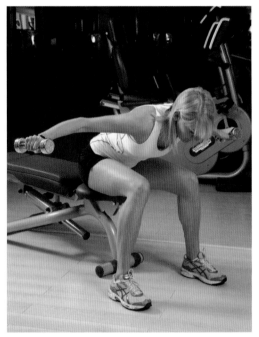

Targets
The upper and middle back.

Method
- Sit on a chair, or the end of a bench, knees bent with feet hip-width apart.
- Bend forwards at the waist, and hold dumb-bells behind your calves, palms facing inwards

- Exhale and lift arms out until your elbows are level with your shoulders.
- Inhale and slowly return to start position.

Training tip
Lower the dumbbells with control to make the exercise as effective as possible.

AB CRUNCH

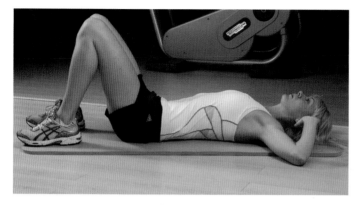

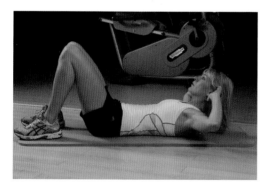

Targets
The abdominal muscles.

Method
- Lie on your back on the floor, feet and knees hip-width apart.
- Place your hands by your ears and breathe in to prepare.
- Exhale and draw your abdominals in as you curl your head and shoulders off the floor.
- Inhale to return to the floor.

Training tip
Keep the neck relaxed – and leave enough space to place a tennis ball under your chin. Try to keep the stomach as flat as possible as you curl up. Perform the movement slowly and with control.

OBLIQUE CRUNCH

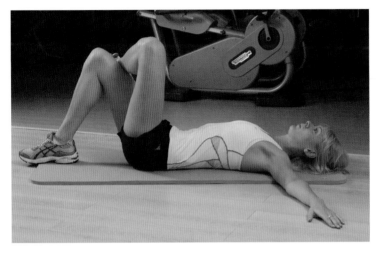

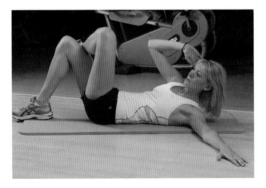

Targets

The oblique muscles in the stomach.

Method

- Lie on your back, feet and knees hip width apart.
- Place your left foot on to your right knee and your right hand by your right ear. Keep your left arm out on the floor at shoulder height, palm down.
- Exhale and curl your right shoulder towards your left hip.
- Inhale back to the centre and repeat.
- Repeat on opposite side.

Training tips

Try to keep your hips still and abdominals flat. Move the shoulder towards the hip rather than the elbow.

REVERSE CRUNCH

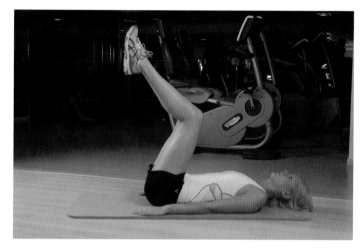

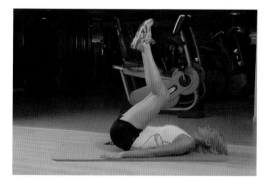

Targets
The abdominal muscles.

Method
- Lie on your back, hands by your sides, and lift legs into the air, feet above the hips.
- Exhale and contract abs to curl your pelvis towards your ribs in a controlled fashion.
- Inhale and to control back to start position.

Training tips
Do not swing the legs or use momentum; a small controlled movement is required. Keep your head down throughout the exercise.

Planning a resistance training programme for your body shape

When planning a resistance programme, you need to go for a whole-body approach – targeting all your major muscle groups. Aim to take into account the following:

- Balance – work opposing muscle groups where possible – for example, abs, then back, biceps, then triceps.
- Variety – try to keep your routines varied and try different weights, or use a flex band as an alternative and change your exercises every 6–8 weeks. This will avoid over-use injury, prevent boredom, and will challenge all your muscles and keep shaping you up.
- Control – try not to rush your exercises. Use slow, controlled movements, especially during the lowering phase.
- Intensity – increase the intensity each sixth workout. This will overload your muscles; this is crucial in order to progress your body shaping. Either add an extra set, more reps or more weight.

SAMPLE PROGRAMMES

'Apples' need to maximise their fat-burning potential and build lean muscle tissue to fire up their metabolism, so compound (multi-muscle) moves are a must. For the following exercises, build up to 3 sets of 12–15 reps with a light weight and progress to a medium weight after 6–8 weeks. Train twice per week.

Sample 1	Sample 2
Warm-up	Warm-up
Walking lunges	Squat with shoulder press
Exercise ball squats	Exercise ball glute raise
Chest press	Upright row
Plie squat with lateral raise	Reverse flye
Triceps dips	Oblique curls
Back extension	Press-ups
Ab curls	Biceps curls
Reverse curls	Exercise ball ab curls

'Pears' need to work on an all-over body programme even though they may feel that they should focus on the lower body. Lifting weights with the upper body will build definition into the shoulders to balance proportions, and remember the more lean muscle you have, the more fat you will burn! So ensure you follow a well-rounded programme, working towards 3 sets of 8–12 repetitions with a medium weight twice per week – once you are sufficiently conditioned.

Sample 1	Sample 2
Warm-up	Warm-up
Squat with shoulder press	Side lunge with wood chop
Plie squat with lateral raise	Press-up
Chest press	Walking lunge
Reverse lunge	Upright row
Triceps dip	Exercise ball glute raise
Biceps curl	Oblique crunch
Ab curls	Ab curls
Reverse curls	Pilates side leg series

Celery shapes need an all-over toning programme. This should focus on the waist line for curves, and build some shape in the shoulders and bottom. To build definition, aim for a weight that fatigues the muscle across 3 sets of 8–12 reps. Once you have conditioned the body, if you are looking for more lean muscle gain, then move on to a heavier weight and do 8–10 reps. Do two to three workouts a week.

Sample 1	Sample 2
Walking lunge	Ball squat
Squat	Reverse lunge
Press-up	Exercise ball chest press
Exercise ball glute raise	Shoulder press
Triceps dips	Reverse flye
Bicep curls	Ab crunch
Oblique crunch	Upright row
Reverse crunch	Oblique crunch

The 'hourglass' needs to keep her curves under control, and may need to tone up her back although her shoulders are usually already good. The arms should be toned, but without building up too much definition, so go for more repetitions with a light weight. Her thighs and bottom should be challenged in order to keep proportions in balance, so add extra resistance by holding dumbbells when squatting and lunging, for example. Build up to 3 sets of 8–12 reps.

Sample 1	Sample 2
Warm-up	Warm-up
Plie squat with lateral raise	Walking lunge
Reverse lunge	Side lunge with wood chop
Press-up	Reverse flye
Biceps curl	Chest press
Triceps dips	Ab curls
Oblique curls	Plank
Back extension	Reverse curls

All body shapes should stretch following their resistance workouts (*see* page 32). Try to focus on the muscle groups you have worked on.

Check page 116–7 to see Lucy's 'before and after' case study!

Pilates

Pilates is a form of resistance training. It can be done daily if required, as opposed to resistance training (that I recommend be done a maximum of three times per week). All Pilates exercises are suitable for all body shapes, although a few may be of more benefit to some, and I highlight these where relevant.

On the following pages, I have provided a selection of exercises that you can do any time, any place, anywhere! You could even add them to the end of your CV or resistance workouts, or do a half-hour Pilates session on your days off. Some of the abdominal exercises, such as the 100, or the criss-cross, can replace your ab curls and other core training in your resistance programme to add variety.

You may have heard that Pilates is excellent for posture and core (abdominal) strength, but it is also fantastic for toning the thighs and lifting the bottom. It is, however, important to apply the following principles:

- Concentration – clear your mind and focus on each and every movement. Stay aware of your body.
- Breathing – Pilates uses lateral (sideways) breathing. Breathe in deep and wide, expanding the ribs to the back and sides; as you exhale, close your ribs downwards and 'soften' your breastbone down. Try this standing in front of a mirror: keep the shoulders relaxed and watch the ribs move in and out to the sides.
- Centring – as you exhale, draw up through the pelvic floor, and draw your navel back towards the spine – 'tightening your girdle'.
- Alignment – make sure your joints are aligned and your posture is correct for each exercise. This will become second nature with practice.
- Relaxation – as with concentration, try to stay relaxed and 'in the moment'. Keep your movements light and fluid.
- Flowing movement – control your movements, and let them flow with your breath. Move your body without strain, lengthening the limbs away from your centre.
- Stamina – build up the exercises slowly, and challenge your stability as you hold positions to build up your stamina. The strong core you can develop will give you great strength, control and stamina through all your other forms of exercise.
- Co-ordination – co-ordinate your alignment, your breathing and centring with your movements.

Pilates exercises

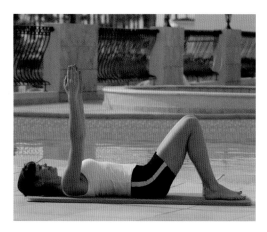

SCISSOR ARMS

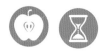

- Lie on your back, feet and knees hip-width apart, and 'float' your hands to point directly upwards.
- Inhale to prepare, exhale, and scissor one arm reaching up behind you and the other towards your feet.
- Inhale back to the centre, exhale in opposite direction.
- Try not to arch your back or let your ribs lift off the floor as you move.

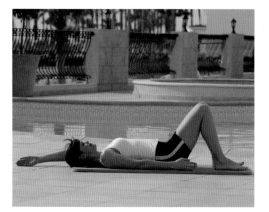

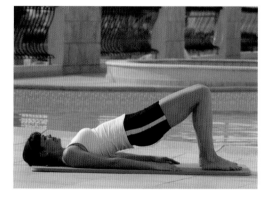

SHOULDER BRIDGE

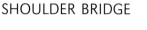
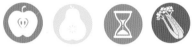

- Lie on your back, knees bent and your feet hip-width apart.
- Exhale as you roll one vertebrae at a time off the floor until your hips are in the air, making a line with your shoulders and knees.
- Inhale to remain in the bridge, keeping knees, hips and shoulders in a line.
- Exhale to return one vertebrae at a time to the floor.

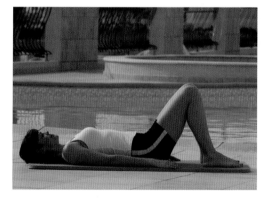

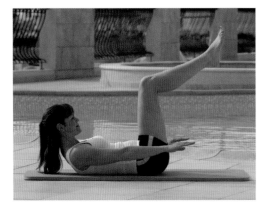

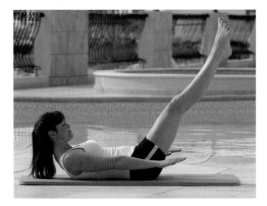

PILATES 100

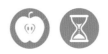

- Lie on your back, contract your abs, and bring both knees in, so that your lower legs are parallel to the ground and your thighs at right angles to it.
- Exhale and lift your head, shoulders and arms off the floor.
- Straighten legs, and begin to beat your arms as if pressing down on springs.
- Inhale for 5 arm beats and exhale for 5 arm beats, building up to 100 beats.

Training tips

Keep your abdominals contracted throughout, and do not let your back arch. Beginners should keep their knees bent. As you progress, gradually straighten the legs. Advanced exercisers should lower straight legs towards the floor.

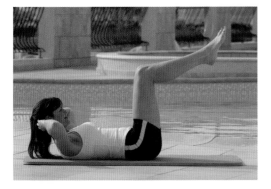

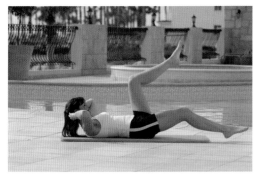

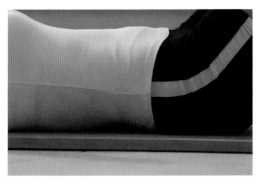

PILATES TOE TAPS

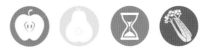

- Lie on your back and lift one leg at a time until your knee is above your hip and bent to 90 degrees.
- Place your fingertips behind your ears, and flex head and shoulders forwards.
- Exhale to lower one foot towards the floor, inhale to return.
- Keep your head and shoulders lifted.

Training tips

As you progress, straighten your leg out as you lower it. Only lower the leg as far as you can while keeping your stomach flat and while maintaining the natural curvature of your spine. As you progress, straighten each leg out as you lower it. Ensure you keep your stomach flat and neutral spine as shown in picture.

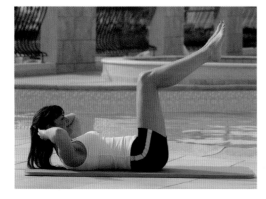

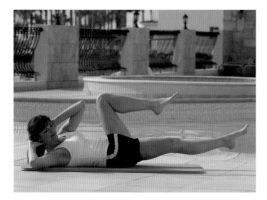

THE PILATES CRISS-CROSS

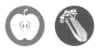

- Lie on your back and connect your navel to your spine as you float one leg at a time up to a right angle.
- Place your fingers behind your ears and keep your elbows wide, then exhale to curl head and shoulders up.
- Exhale and peel left shoulder across towards your right hip as you extend the right leg out – as low as you can while keeping stomach flat and spine's natural curves.
- Inhale back to centre and exhale in opposite direction.
- Do 10 slow repetitions followed by 10 fast, but controlled, repetitions.

Training tips

Try to keep your stomach flat throughout, and move in a controlled manner – don't let your hips rock as you move. Imagine you are folding your shoulder towards the opposite hip.

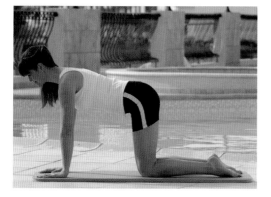

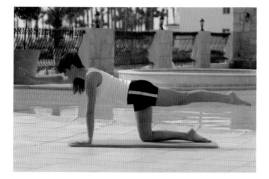

SWIMMING

- Kneel on all fours. Keep your knees under your hips and hands under your shoulders while still maintaining the natural curve of your spine.
- Inhale to prepare and exhale, drawing your navel to your spine as you lengthen your opposite arm and leg away from you until they lift off the floor.
- Inhale to return to centre.
- Exhale to lengthen opposite side limbs away.

Training tips

Keep your torso still throughout. Imagine that there are four glasses of water sitting on the four corners of your back and try not to spill a drop! Keep your head and neck in line with your spine.

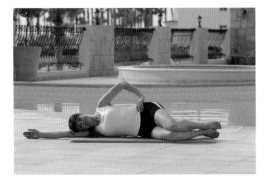

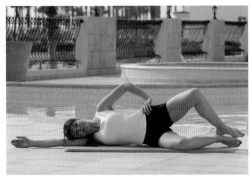

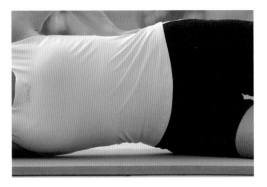

SIDE LYING LEGS SERIES: PART 1

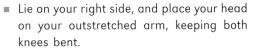

- Lie on your right side, and place your head on your outstretched arm, keeping both knees bent.
- Exhale to open left knee like a clam shell; your feet stay together on the floor.
- Inhale to close.

Training tips

Keep your navel drawn into your spine, and do not let your hips roll back as you open the knee.

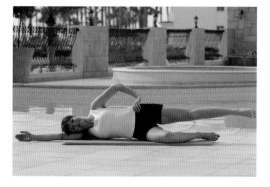

SIDE LYING LEGS SERIES: PART 2

- Lie on your right side, head on outstretched arm, right leg bent and left leg out straight.
- Keep your waist off the floor as you lift your left foot to hip height, exhaling as you do so.
- Inhale to return to hip height.

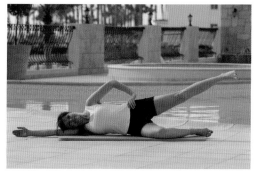

SIDE LYING LEGS SERIES: PART 3

- Lie on your right side, left leg bent for stability, right leg out straight at hip height.
- Draw circles in the air with left foot in each direction.

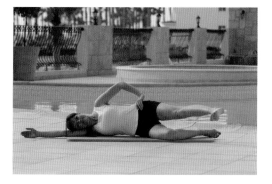

Training tip
Keep your waist lengthened off the floor (*see* photo bottom-left), and maintain navel to spine connection throughout.

Repeat entire side lying leg series on other side.

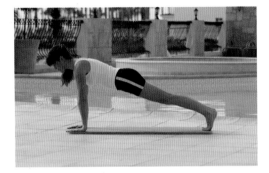

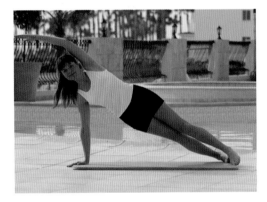

THE PLANK AND SIDE PLANK SERIES

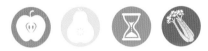

- Place your hands under your shoulders, keep your back straight, and extend your legs out behind you, while supporting your body weight on your hands and toes. Hold for 10 to 30 seconds depending on your fitness.
- Keep your abdominals engaged as you lift your right arm out to the right side, turning your hips slowly to the right until you are in a side plank.
- Rotate hips and arm back to the centre into plank position and repeat on the left side.

Training tips

This is quite advanced, so stick with the first position until you are strong enough to turn and balance. Keep head in line with the spine, and maintain its natural curves. Do not allow your bottom to poke up in the air!

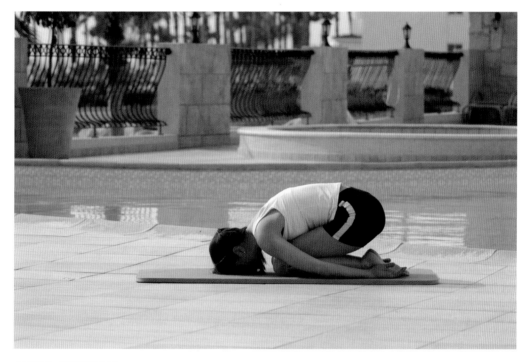

SHELL STRETCH

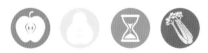

- From the plank, move into a kneeling position, then lower your bottom back on to your heels, with your forehead down on to the floor.
- Rest your fingertips down by your toes and allow your shoulders to relax.

- Breathe deeply, imagining your spine lengthening and broadening with each exhale.
- Stay for six breaths.

Yoga

Like Pilates, yoga can be an effective form of resistance exercise and I have dedicated a separate section to this discipline.

Yoga in its traditional form is more a way of life than a system of exercise, and the asanas (exercises) are wonderful for flexibility, strength and stamina. Yoga has been practised for thousands of years and there are four different paths – 'Jnana yoga', the study of ancient scriptures, 'karma yoga', selfless service or doing good for no reward, 'Bhakti yoga', which includes practices such as chanting and the repetition of mantras, and 'Raja yoga', which is based on a practical system of concentration and control of the mind through asanas, breathing and meditation.

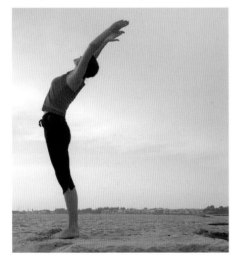

Different styles of yoga class

- Hatha yoga – Hatha yoga is based on posture work and relaxation, and is found in most general, traditional yoga classes, which should be suitable for beginners and all levels.
- Astanga yoga – Astanga yoga tends to be more dynamic and challenging. You have to move quickly between postures.
- Bikram yoga – Bikram yoga is very popular right now. It is performed in a very hot room, and is not suitable for the very overweight or unfit.

Yoga is a huge subject and there are hundreds of asanas. It can't easily be summed up in a short chapter, so for the purpose of this book I have provided examples of asanas that will have a positive effect on your body shape, and your overall mental and physical health.

For further yoga information, check out your local gym or search online for a qualified local instructor and yoga organisations.

Selected yoga exercises

SUN SALUTATIONS

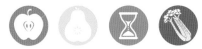

Sun salutations are a wonderful way to warm up the body in readiness for any exercise routine. They can be performed slowly and meditatively, or faster for a dynamic warm-up. There are many variations; here is a very traditional series, which can be performed 6–12 times:

1 Stand tall and strong, with feet together and your hands in prayer position.
2 Inhale and stretch your arms up over your head, alongside your ears. Arch back from the waist and push your hips forward.

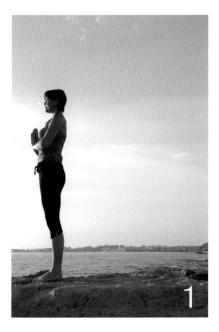

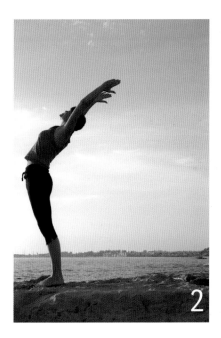

3   Exhale and fold forward from the waist. Stretch your arms forwards, bring your hands down to the floor by your feet (bend your knees for leg flexibility) and tuck your head into your knees.

5   Hold your breath as you step the left foot back and place it alongside the right to form a plank with your body. Keep your stomach muscles tight and your back flat and strong.

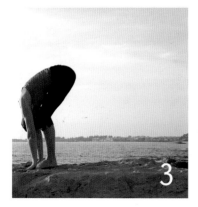

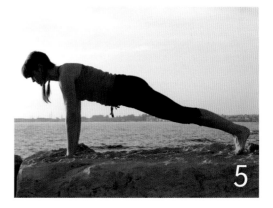

4   Inhale as you step the right leg back as far as possible and drop the right knee.

6   Exhale and lower your knees, chest and chin to the floor.

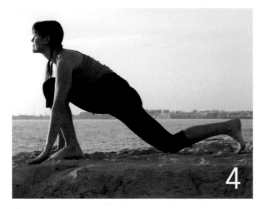

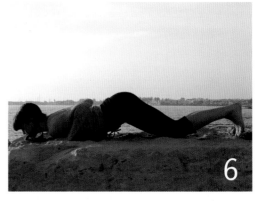

7 Inhale and slide your hips forward, arching your chest, head and chin up into the 'cobra' position.

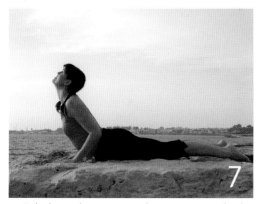

8 Exhale and press your hips up towards the ceiling, keeping your hands and feet still, forming an inverted 'v'.

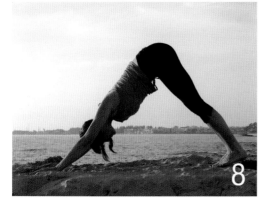

9 Inhale and step your right foot forwards between your hands, dropping your knee to the floor and lifting your chest.

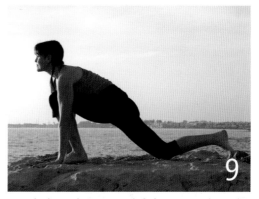

10 Exhale and step your left foot up to the right, placing your hands either side and tucking your head into your knees.

11 Inhale, stretch back up to start position (step 2), and continue sequence stepping back with the left leg.

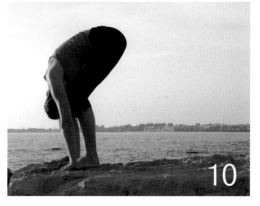

THE DOLPHIN (FANTASTIC FOR ARMS AND SHOULDERS, BUT NOT FOR BEGINNERS)

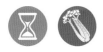

1 Kneel and sit back on your heels, and place your elbows on the floor. Interlock your fingers together in front of you (*see* photo below), keeping your elbows shoulder-width apart (measure the correct distance by clasping each hand around the opposite elbow.

2 Without moving the elbows, lift your bottom up until your weight is on your elbows and feet, with your bottom making the point of a triangle (*see* photo right).

3 Rock your body forwards, bringing your chin towards the floor in front of your hands (*see* photo bottom right).

4 Rock the body back, pushing back with your arms, and rock back and forth several times.

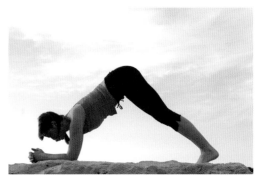

5 Rest your bottom on your heels and your forehead on the floor – this is known as 'child's pose'.

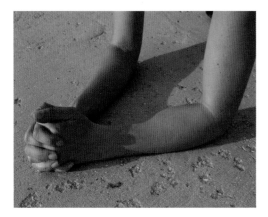

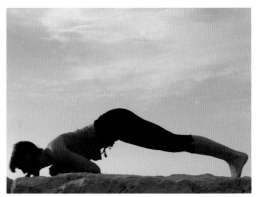

THE BRIDGE – BEGINNER'S VERSION

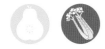

- Lie on your back, knees bent and feet close to your bottom, hands by your sides.
- Raise your hips as high as possible by squeezing your buttocks.
- Keep your knees in line with your hips and hold for several breaths.

THE TREE – FANTASTIC FOR FOCUSING THE MIND

- Stand straight, balancing on your left leg.
- Bend your right leg and place the sole of your right foot on the inside of your left thigh, or your lower leg if you do not have the flexibility required (you can use your hand to help place your foot on to the thigh).
- Focus your eyes on a point straight ahead, bring your hands together in the prayer position in front of your chest, and find your balance.
- Keep the palms together and raise your hands up over your head.
- Stand and breathe gently for 30 seconds to a minute before repeating on the other leg.

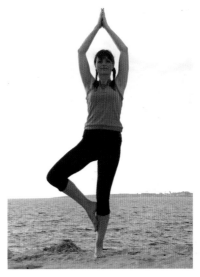

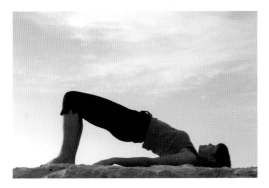

7 SPORTS TRAINING AND EXERCISE CLASSES

Sports and team games are a great way to have fun and make friends while shaping up. Below are some great reasons why.

Sports

TENNIS

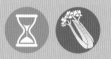

Tennis is a fantastic way to shape up your lower and upper body and, depending on your standard, can be a good calorie fat burner. Tennis can define your upper body, but if you play regularly, resistance train your non-hitting arm as well to promote symmetrical body development.

NETBALL

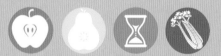

This is a good all-round activity, as it involves short bursts of running and lots of twisting, throwing and jumping, depending on your team position. Most netball clubs will also do some general fitness work.

WOMEN'S RUGBY

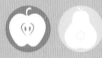

Women's rugby is becoming more popular, and is a great game for larger women, although there is a place in rugby for all body shapes provided you have a reasonable base level of fitness. If you join a local team, your training will give you a great all-over condition. If you play, depending on your position, you will develop strength, power and muscle definition.

WOMEN'S FOOTBALL

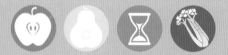

Football is the fastest growing sport for women. It's got the aerobic and anaerobic benefits of rugby and will build strong, shapely legs.

SQUASH

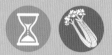

Squash is a challenging game, just like an interval training session with lots of bursts of activity. It's an ideal challenge for a 'celery' or 'hourglass' looking to improve CV fitness in a team environment.

ATHLETICS

From the lean, muscled physique of the sprinters and jumpers, to the slighter middle- and long-distance runners and the bigger throwers, there's an event for all body shapes.

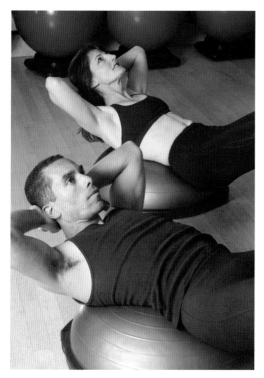

Exercise classes

There are now many different exercise classes available to women, from boxing to ballet. Find the best classes for your shape below.

AEROBICS

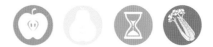

This is good general cardiovascular exercise that burns lots of calories. Beginners' aerobics is a great place to get started on your exercise routine, although some co-ordination is required!

AQUAROBICS

Aquarobics is an aerobics class performed in the pool, and this makes it very suitable for beginners, and overweight 'apples' and 'pears', as the water supports your weight. The water also provides resistance, so while good for muscle toning, is also kind on your joints.

BOXING CLASSES

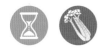

Both boxing and boxing-based aerobic classes are great calorie burners, developing CV fitness and all-over tone. Box-aerobics is essentially an aerobics class with a boxing theme, including punches and kicking, in a choreographed routine. Boxercise is a non-contact sparring option, while Padbox can be done one on one with a suitably qualified personal trainer. Training at a boxing club is likely to incorporate pad work, skipping and body conditioning – adding lots of variety to your training.

For boxing and derivative workouts a reasonable level of fitness is required, and some pre-conditioning work is advised.

CIRCUIT TRAINING

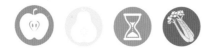

Circuit training is a great class for all body shapes (although overweight 'apples' and 'pears' should be mindful of the jumping exercises that a class might contain). Classes begin with a general aerobic warm-up, followed by a combination of challenges to be sustained for intervals. All body parts should get a workout, unless you choose a specific upper or lower body circuit class. The benefit of circuit classes is that they combine CV work with toning and flexibility. They're also great for the time-pressed individual as they provide nearly all types of fitness in one workout.

DANCE CLASSES

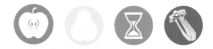

There are hundreds of fun dance classes, salsa, jazz, ballet – to name but a few. Not only can dance be a great aerobic challenge, it can work wonders for flexibility and posture. Good co-ordination is obviously a prerequisite! Dance classes can also be a fun social activity that doesn't feel like exercise, and can add variety into your routine.

If you are not used to exercise, doing some exercises to strengthen your knees and ankles is advisable (*see* pre-conditioning on page 37).

EXERCISE CLASS WITH WEIGHTS

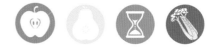

Weights are used to tone the muscles and have an added CV aspect. This class is great for all body shapes as it will give definition without bulk due to the high repetitions used and the low weight. Check your instructor is certified as technique is crucial to prevent injury, and don't be afraid to change to lighter weights if fatigue causes your form to suffer.

INDOOR CYCLING CLASSES

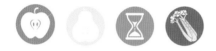

Indoor cycling is a great fat-burning CV class suitable for all body shapes, although it requires a good level of starting fitness, and so is not suited to very overweight or out-of-condition women. A cycle class can include some upper body work (on and off the bike) as well as interval training and hill climbing, and is great for people wanting to challenge their fitness.

MILITARY-STYLE WORKOUTS

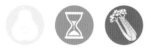

Military-type sessions are similar to circuit training and involve some running, jumping, squatting and sit-ups and so on. I would therefore not recommend them for an overweight 'apple'. If you have a reasonable level of fitness, and you have pre-conditioned, then this is a good option to push you on to the next level. Fitter pear shapes can get a good interval training session, and celery shapes will appreciate the muscle toning and great abdominal workout. These workouts are to be avoided if injured, pregnant or very overweight. They are great in the summer as often the classes take place in the open air.

STEP AEROBICS

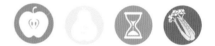

Step classes can be quite challenging. The class requires co-ordination, and provides a good fat-burning CV workout; it is particularly challenging for the lower body. It is not suitable for complete beginners.

8 PREGNANCY AND MENOPAUSE

Pregnancy and post-natal exercise

The nine months of pregnancy are a unique time, and your body will undergo many changes. It is not the right time to embark on a new fitness campaign if you have never previously exercised, so, if possible, you should try to work on your health and fitness prior to conception.

For those of you already exercising regularly,

provided your GP has given you the all-clear, there is no reason why you should not continue to exercise as long as you moderate your routine progressively.

During pregnancy your body produces the hormone relaxin and it is important to take this into account when exercising or stretching. Relaxin increases elasticity in the ligaments in order to allow the pelvis to accommodate the pregnancy and birth. This means that your

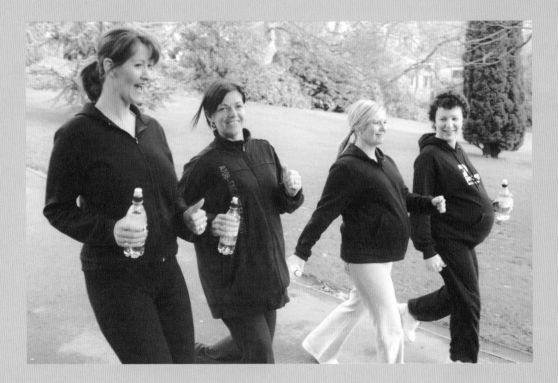

joints become much more vulnerable and unstable. Stretching exercises should therefore be approached with caution and you should always seek advice from an expert if you are unsure. You should also be aware that it will take 5 to 6 months after birth for relaxin to leave the body.

Yoga and Pilates are both excellent forms of exercise during pregnancy, as they are controlled and gentle, and they will help with the breathing required for giving birth. Pilates is excellent for training and strengthening the deep pelvic floor muscles, and it is worth practising this before, during and after pregnancy.

The importance of specific nutrition during pregnancy

Calorie restriction is not advisable when pregnant – you'll need to eat more as you are eating for two (or more!). It's recommended that from the middle of the second trimester onwards that you consume an additional 200–300 calories a day.

It's key that you and your developing baby receive the best nutrients. To this end, carbohydrates are very important; not only will they provide you with energy, but they'll also supply your growing baby with placental and foetal glucose. Your protein consumption should be 75g to 100g per day. Most women's weight will increase by 10–15kg during pregnancy.

Remaining hydrated is equally important, so aim for 2–3 litres of water or fruit juice a day.

Table 11 Selected recommended vitamin and mineral consumption during pregnancy	
Vitamin/mineral	**Recommended daily intake**
Calcium	1000–1200mg
Iron	30mg
Folic acid	800mcg (micrograms)

You should also ensure that you are getting enough B vitamins; if you supplement, you should be aiming for 20mcg of vitamin B12, 200mg of vitamin B6, and 250mg of magnesium.

Post-natal exercise

Post-natal exercise is very important and will help your body regain its posture, strength and tone, but you should never rush into a new regime. Your body will take time to settle back into shape, and weight loss should not be rushed – particularly if you are breastfeeding, as adequate nutrition and calories are very important.

Once you decide the time is right to start thinking of exercise, and your doctor has given you the all-clear, then there are a few key points to bear in mind:

- The hormone relaxin – this will still affect the body after delivery, so be aware of your joint stability.
- Posture – your spine and pelvis will have been under a lot of strain, and will most likely need to be re-trained back to a healthy neutral position that maintains the natural curves of your upper and lower back. Pilates exercises should help you learn how to find and keep a healthy neutral position which you should focus on maintaining throughout your exercises.
- Abdominals – some of the abdominal muscles separate during pregnancy to leave space for the baby, and the rectus abdominus (the large muscle down the front of your stomach) muscle can lengthen by up to 8 inches! So it is really of no surprise that your stomach will appear different. However, around six weeks after delivery, the separated muscle should have returned to about a two fingers' width.

I have provided examples of some gentle exercises that you can do after delivery to encourage the muscle to come together. Try them as soon as you feel able.

ABDOMINAL ENGAGING

- Lie on your back, knees bent and hip-width apart, neutral spine (neither flat nor arched).
- Exhale and draw your tummy button in towards your spine, flattening the abs while keeping the pelvis still.
- Inhale and release.

PELVIC TILTS

- Lie on your back as above, with your back in neutral position.
- Exhale as you draw your tummy button in and tilt your pelvis until your lower back sinks towards the floor.
- Inhale and release your back to return to neutral spine position.

Menopause

The menopause can be a difficult time for women. It represents the stage in life where the ovaries cease to produce oestrogen, and stop producing an egg each month. Many women may experience a loss of control, feelings of depression, and erratic mood swings.

Physiologically, the changes associated with the menopause may increase the risk of heart disease and osteoporosis, and emotionally a woman may feel she is losing her femininity. However, nowadays there is no need to worry as there is so much information to hand, and countless supplements and creams to help you through the process; hormone treatments can be prescribed where needed.

One of the most powerful things that you can do for yourself at this time, regardless of any other treatment you may follow, is exercise and lift weights. Not only will this help with your body shape, it will assist the maintenance of bone density, and bolster against heart disease. Crucially, exercise will be very beneficial emotionally for reducing stress and give you more of a sense of control.

Many women notice that their bodies becomes slacker and fatter as they age. After the menopause many see their mid-section widen as they take on a new (unwanted) body shape due to changes in metabolism. Diet alone will not be enough to tackle this situation, and you will need to focus on boosting your metabolism by building lean muscle tissue with resistance work and blasting calories with regular CV work.

9 TRAINING PLANNING AND THE MENTAL APPROACH

I have found that women often don't work out to a systematic training plan, and because of this their training efforts are not optimised. Regardless of your body shape, you won't get the most from it unless your workout is relevant to you, and you have a focused training plan. In this chapter I show you how to plan your workouts to achieve your best ever shape.

Don't be afraid to ask for help

Women often feel intimidated in the gym, and may feel nervous about asking for help. But in order to get great results, you *should* ask for assistance. Gym instructors and personal trainers are only too willing to help – and it's their job to assist and supervise us. Also, asking for help is a good way to make gym buddies, and to pick up new tips. Personal trainers and gym instructors can motivate and ensure that you work out safely and effectively. In our

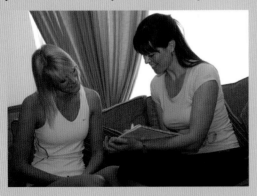

increasingly time-poor lives, they can offer a way to maximise gym time, so that it is not wasted.

Personal trainers

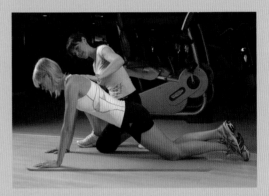

A weekly session with a personal trainer can keep you focused and on course to reach your goals. They can monitor progress and tweak training so that you continue to improve. Even the most experienced trainer can still learn something. If you want a personal trainer, make sure that he or she has the right personality for you – you can try a few out! Obviously they should be relevantly qualified and insured.

Planning your training

If you intend to plan your own workouts, you should follow these steps. However, if you are new to training or are returning after a long lay-off I would recommend that you book at least a couple of sessions with a personal trainer.

Pulling it all together – constructing a training plan for your body shape

STEP 1: ANALYSE YOUR BODY TYPE AND SHAPE

Using the information provided in this book, you should be able to determine your body type and your current body shape and whether, for example, you need to lose fat, tone up or increase lean muscle. Once you have done this, you are in an informed position to plan your training.

STEP 2: SET SOME GOALS

Without goals you will not be able to line up your training. Goals are important motivators. You'll need short- and long-term ones. The former will act as stepping stones on the way to achieving the latter.

You should use the SMART goal-setting principles. Basically your goals should be:

- Specific
- Measurable
- Achievable
- Realistic
- Targeted.

Example:
Body shape: apple
Training goal: to lose weight by Xkg (specify your own realistic target weight loss) and to fall within acceptable BMI levels in four months. This will be specific to you and your starting weight (acceptable weight loss at the outset of training programme is 1–2lb a week (0.5–1kg)).

STEP 3: CONSTRUCTING YOUR TRAINING PLAN

A simple way to plan your training if you want to do it yourself is to use the training pyramid concept. Basically, this model builds increased levels of fitness on previous levels of fitness as you progress to your goal – the apex of the pyramid.

The training pyramid can be applied to any fitness or sports training target. Each phase should be long enough (usually between 6 and 18 weeks) to allow your body to optimally adapt without stagnation setting in. When planning your training, allow at least 3 to 6 months to reach the top of the pyramid and achieve your goal/goals.

Training tip

To get the most from your training you need to adopt a cyclical approach, emphasising different training aspects, components and variables at different times to achieve progressive and optimum results. The training pyramid on page 112 is ideal in this respect.

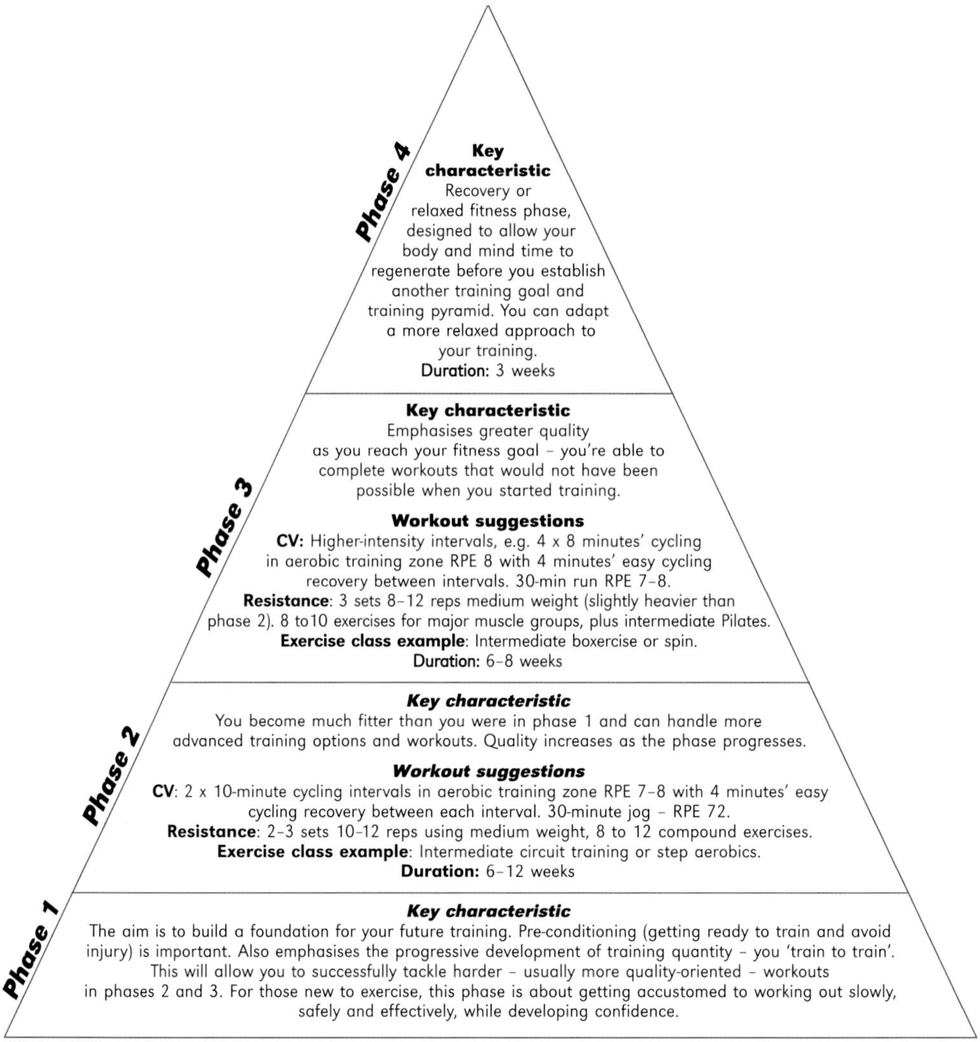

Phase 4

Key characteristic
Recovery or relaxed fitness phase, designed to allow your body and mind time to regenerate before you establish another training goal and training pyramid. You can adapt a more relaxed approach to your training.
Duration: 3 weeks

Phase 3

Key characteristic
Emphasises greater quality as you reach your fitness goal – you're able to complete workouts that would not have been possible when you started training.

Workout suggestions
CV: Higher-intensity intervals, e.g. 4 x 8 minutes' cycling in aerobic training zone RPE 8 with 4 minutes' easy cycling recovery between intervals. 30-min run RPE 7–8.
Resistance: 3 sets 8–12 reps medium weight (slightly heavier than phase 2). 8 to 10 exercises for major muscle groups, plus intermediate Pilates.
Exercise class example: Intermediate boxercise or spin.
Duration: 6–8 weeks

Phase 2

Key characteristic
You become much fitter than you were in phase 1 and can handle more advanced training options and workouts. Quality increases as the phase progresses.

Workout suggestions
CV: 2 x 10-minute cycling intervals in aerobic training zone RPE 7–8 with 4 minutes' easy cycling recovery between each interval. 30-minute jog – RPE 72.
Resistance: 2–3 sets 10–12 reps using medium weight, 8 to 12 compound exercises.
Exercise class example: Intermediate circuit training or step aerobics.
Duration: 6–12 weeks

Phase 1

Key characteristic
The aim is to build a foundation for your future training. Pre-conditioning (getting ready to train and avoid injury) is important. Also emphasises the progressive development of training quantity – you 'train to train'. This will allow you to successfully tackle harder – usually more quality-oriented – workouts in phases 2 and 3. For those new to exercise, this phase is about getting accustomed to working out slowly, safely and effectively, while developing confidence.

Fig. 9.1 *The training pyramid*

The training variables

The training variables of quantity, quality, duration, intensity and rest are fundamental to constructing a progressive training plan – they will inform and shape your individual workouts and your overall plan.

- Quantity refers to the amount of training done either in a particular workout or as part of a particular training phase. It can be measured by the number of kilometres covered for CV training, or total weight lifted, repetitions or sets completed for weight training.
- Quality usually reflects the intensity of a workout. A low-quality workout may involve an easy-pace run; a high-quality one will involve a series of near flat-out intervals. You should balance the quality of your workouts over your training plan to avoid overtraining and potential injury.
- Duration applies to the length of a workout and is therefore more applicable to CV training than weight training. In this respect, it references the length of a workout or particular aspect of it (such as an interval) and is inextricably linked to quantity and quality.
- Frequency refers to the number of weekly or other period workouts.
- Rest is just as important as training – this is when all the benefits accrue. Without sufficient rest adaptive processes will not take place. Rest days, rest periods and the carefully constructed use of light, medium and hard workouts are all crucial to the balanced training plan.

Progressive overload and adaptation

Progressive overload is perhaps the key principle of training if you want to get the most from your shape. Put simply, if you don't progressively overload you won't improve your fitness whatever your body shape.

However, you should not start off at a too intense level as this will lead to disappointment when you can't, for example, complete as many weights reps as you think you should, or, at worst, this could lead to injury. Begin at a low intensity and allow enough time between sessions for recovery. In time your body will adapt – you'll find lifting the weights easier. At this point you can then increase the intensity to produce further increases in fitness. If there is no progression, then your fitness level will plateau.

Table 12 Example of a progressive overload programme (particularly suited to those new to exercise)				
Week	1 and 2	3 and 4	5 and 6	7 and 8
Reps and sets	2 sets x 5 reps	3 sets x 5 reps	3 sets x 8 reps	3 sets x 10 reps
Frequency	2 x per week	2 x per week	2 x per week	2 x per week

Table 12 shows a simple volume progression. The goal at the start is to learn the exercises correctly. In this example, you perform only 2 sets x 5 reps twice a week for weeks 1 and 2, to ensure the muscles and tendons involved in the exercise are not overloaded too much too soon. During weeks 3 and 4 you complete 50 per cent more reps by adding another set (3 x 5). Over the next 4 weeks, you build up to 3 sets x 10 reps, which is three times the original quantity.

Training tip

Don't become overly preoccupied with how your body is looking; rather, relax into your workouts and, over time, the changes will happen. If you become too concerned and stressed you may over-train or fail to appreciate the gains you have already made.

Over-training

Although exercise is good for you, there are times when too much of it can have a detrimental effect and potentially lead to over-training syndrome (OTS). A carefully constructed training programme incorporating sufficient rest and recovery should avoid OTS. But if you do suffer from some of the symptoms in the box below, and have been in hard training for a while, you could be suffering from OTS. If you think that you are, take at least a week off training, before returning to your workouts, and then at a lower level than when you stopped.

OVER-TRAINING SYMPTOMS

- A lack of desire to want to train.
- Continuously feeling fatigued and listless.
- Decreased maximal heart rate.
- Greater susceptibility to illness – particularly upper respiratory tract infections
- Mood swings.
- Feelings of anxiousness and stress.
- An increase in resting heart rate.*
- Sleep problems.
- Lack of appetite.

* Resting heart rate (RHR) should be taken a few minutes after waking; an increase above 'normal' can indicate that you have not fully recovered from your previous workouts or are stressed. If your RHR has increased, then you should either take the day off from training or perform an easy workout.

Lifestyle – you can find the time to work out

Fitting in workouts and eating healthily can be a challenge, considering all the other constraints and distractions we have in our lives. However, there are many ways to do this. Here are some really simple suggestions for fitting workouts into your daily routines:

- Run or cycle to work.
- Get a joint gym membership for you and your partner.
- Take up an active weekend hobby like mountain biking.
- Enter a local fun run (or even marathon) and train for it.

Any of these and other ideas will put exercise into your lifestyle – in some cases, without you even realising it.

Daily activity will also have an effect on your calorie expenditure, so try to move as much as possible – take the stairs instead of the lift, walk the kids to school instead of driving, get off the bus a stop early, and run up and down the stairs several times a day. Every bit helps!

Case study and example training programme: Lucy, age 42

Lucy was concerned about a thickening mid-section, although she was typically a classic pear shape with excess fat on her hips and lower body. She had a reasonable level of fitness, and was active most days – walking for 15 minutes morning and evening, and attending one yoga class per week.

I decided Lucy needed to begin a quality weight training routine in order to boost her metabolism and define her body. We incorporated CV work in her warm-up, and tried to raise her heart rate in between some sets with skipping and step-ups. We trained at her home, using dumbbells, an exercise ball, a weighted medicine ball and a skipping rope.

Week 1 – repeat twice
20 minutes' fast walk
2 x 10 walking lunges
15 medicine ball squats and
    medicine ball chest presses
12 shoulder press
12 medicine ball glute raises
15 ab curls and reverse curls
Pilates side leg series
Stretches

Week 2 – repeat 2–3 times
25 minutes' fast walk
2 x 12 walking lunges
2 x 10 squat with shoulder press
    using medicine ball
1 x 10 press-ups, lateral raises with dumbbells
    and triceps bench dips
Pilates criss-cross
Pilates 100
Stretches

Week 3
15 minutes' fast walk
Step-ups 6 minutes
3 sets 10 medicine ball chest press
2 sets 10 squat with dumbbell shoulder press
2 sets 10 plie squat with lateral raise
1 x 15 ball glute raise
2 x 10 reverse flye
10 back extension
2 x 10 bicep curl
15 ab curls with medicine ball
Stretches

Week 4 – repeat 2–3 times
20 minutes' fast walk with 2 minutes' jog inter-
    vals walking lunges carrying dumbbells
3 x 10 ball squats with dumbbells
3 x 10 medicine ball chest press
3 x 8 tricep bench dips
3 x 10 plie squats with 1 set lateral raise
2 x 10 shoulder press with dumbbells
Plank – hold 12 seconds
Pilates criss-cross and side leg series
Reverse curls
Stretches

This takes you to the end of the first month. Everybody is different – regardless of body shape – so we will all respond differently. Lucy was already quite strong as she had done similar exercise programmes in the past. For the second month we increased the weight slightly and did 3 sets of 12 reps. Lucy found it hard to manage three workouts per week, so I encouraged her to continue with her weekly yoga, and to try to be as active as possible in general life. Lucy's results are shown in Table 13.

Training tip

Many, if not most, women are unhappy with their body shape, or at least a part of their body, but it is important to be positive and believe in the exercise and dietary regime that you are following, whatever your fitness or body-shaping goals. Try to set realistic goals, remember your body type, and work towards being the best you realistically can be. It is equally important not to become disillusioned with how your body shapes up. If you have established realistic training goals and an equally realistic training plan, then you will get results. Yes, certain body shapes will have to work harder than others to achieve their goals, but a great deal is possible. The right training and mental attitude will get results.

Table 13 Lucy's results

	Weight (kg)	Bust (in)	Under bust (in)	Top hip (in)	Bottom hip (in)	Waist (in)	Top thigh (in)	Biceps (in)
Before	63	35.5	29	38	41.5	29.5	23.75	12
After	60	34	28	36.5	38.5	27	22	11

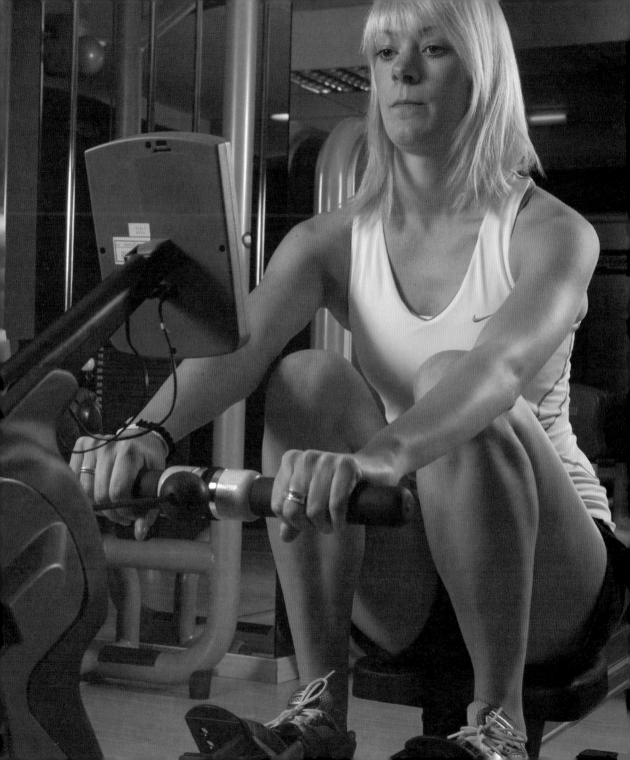

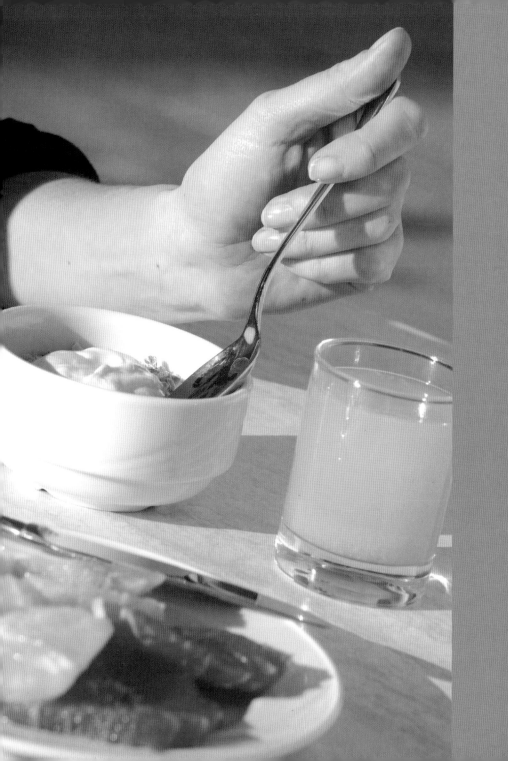

10 NUTRITION FOR YOUR BODY: THE BASICS, MACRO- AND MICRO-NUTRIENTS

As women, we probably have a better idea about the calorie content of food than many guys, and probably begin to count calories as soon as we want to lose fat. However, many of us drastically restrict our food intake – even cutting out whole food groups – in order to attempt to lose weight. This is not a good idea as you may lose out on vital nutrients, and there is a very good chance that your metabolism will slow down, paradoxically leading to a greater chance of weight gain than when calorie restriction is not followed.

In Part 3 of the book I begin the 'energy balance equation'. This will put into context the number of calories you need to lose (or gain), in order to maintain weight. I then consider the main food groups (the macro-nutrients) and explain what vitamins and minerals (the micro-nutrients) and selected supplements can do for you. In the last part of this section the calorie and macro-nutrient content of selected foods are provided to make the process of food selection easier.

Food for life

As women, we tend to be much more aware of food content and labelling than men, as well as becoming increasingly educated about what we are eating. However, do we know what we really should eat? We receive so many mixed messages. There are celebrities telling us how we can be like them if we follow the 'cabbage soup/no carbs/grapefruit' or some other crazy diet! Same 'diets' often have no sound nutritional validity.

In my experience of training and working with women, I have found that a high percentage have a bad relationship with food. They may actually fear food, and view it as the enemy. This is of course silly; no piece of lamb has ever been arrested for GBH! So, I want to provide women with a well-rounded knowledge of food, and how to eat – knowledge that will enable you to get the most from your workouts and all-round body shaping.

Diet

Most women wanting to lose weight start with their diet. Some may not exercise at all or some may exercise as an afterthought, but most will calorie count in one way or another. Now, as previously mentioned, in order to lose fat, calories 'in' need to be less than calories 'out'. You need to create a negative energy balance (*see* energy balance on page 122). Unfortunately, some women become preoccupied with calories *in*, and try to restrict them significantly to speed weight loss. I have had many clients ask me why they have not lost weight when they have only had a bowl of cereal and a bowl of soup all day!

DON'T 'YO-YO' DIET

The answer to the above question is crucial both for health and weight loss. If you drastically restrict your calorie consumption, your body's metabolism can slow to try and conserve calories to prevent starvation. This can set off a very damaging cycle, known as 'yo-yo' dieting, where you diet, lose weight, and then gain weight again as soon as the calorie restriction is lifted. Not only is this physically unhealthy, but it can be psychologically damaging, creating feelings of failure, guilt and even depression.

Another side effect of the 'diets' many women will have experienced is a lack of muscle tone and definition. The generally accepted safe rate of weight loss is 0.5–1kg (1–2lb) per week. Weight loss faster than this can cause a loss of lean muscle tissue, so although the scales read lighter, your body will not have the tightness you desire.

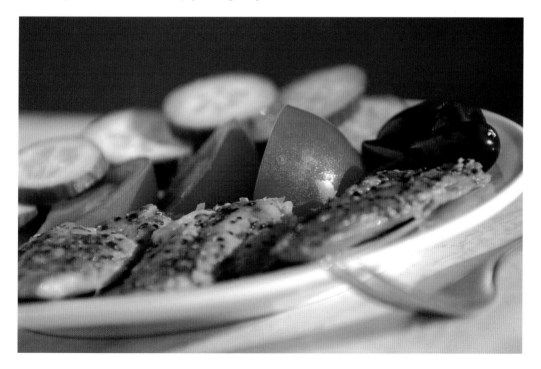

The energy balance equation

Whatever your body shape, it's crucial that you understand the energy balance equation as this will significantly affect the way you shape up. To lose weight, you need to create a negative energy balance – that is, consume fewer calories than those needed to maintain current weight/energy needs (but not, as I have said, excessively). Want to gain muscle tone and shape up? Then you'll probably need to create a positive energy balance – that is, consume more calories to sustain your weight and energy levels. This will enable you to fuel your body to maintain your training and everyday life energy levels and to supply your muscles with the right nutrients to promote increased tone. And to maintain weight you need to match calorie consumption with calorie expenditure – that is, create a balanced energy balance.

Daily calorific requirements

Many food labels now list nutritional information, including guideline daily amounts – for example, calories per day 1600, fat 70g, and salt 5g. These are guidelines only, and are very general. Your age, body type, current shape, fitness level and activity level will all influence the *actual* calories you need on a daily basis. A sedentary, 45-year-old, overweight 'apple' will have very different nutritional and calorific needs than, say, a fit, active 'hourglass' horse trainer.

On page 20 you will find information on how to calculate your daily energy needs, while on page 22 you will find calorie burning figures for selected exercise activities. To this you need to figure in post-exercise calorie burning (EPOC) if you work out regularly, 3–4 times a week, and/or have a physically demanding job (*see* page 52).

Table 14 The energy balance equation

kcal intake	kcal output	Effect on weight	Energy balance
1600	1600	none	balanced
2000	1600	increase	positive
1600	1900	decrease	negative

Note: 'Energy balance' refers to balance between calories consumed and calories expended.

Training tip

In this increasingly technological age numerous gadgets are available to calculate metabolic rate and calorie expenditure.

Heart rate monitors
Many heart rate monitors have calorie counting functions. These use a calculation related to heart rate to estimate calories burned during exercise and everyday activity. These are at most 90 per cent effective (*see* page 54).

Metabolic rate measurement devices
These are worn on the upper arm and record metabolic rate by way of galvanic skin response. They are 100 per cent accurate. Originating from the medical world, they are now becoming increasingly available in the fitness market.

Macro-nutrients

Carbohydrate, fat and protein are 'macro-nutrients' (vitamins and minerals are 'micro-nutrients', *see* page 132). Carbohydrate, fat and protein have very different bodily functions for general health, sports and fitness purposes. Table 15 identifies the energy release from macro-nutrients per gram (in calories). You'll see fat contains more than twice as many calories as carbohydrate and fat.

Fat is high in calories, yet it doesn't provide you with much energy. Hence, too much fat makes you fat!

Carbohydrate and fat are the body's preferred energy sources during exercise. Although protein can also supply energy, this is usually only the result of prolonged CV workouts, when the body's stores of carbohydrate run low. This is why celery shapes and slighter hourglass shapes should be mindful of incorporating too much CV into their workouts if they are after increased muscle size, shape and

Table 15 Energy release from macro-nutrients (kcal)			
Macro-nutrient	**Carbohydrate**	**Fat**	**Protein**
Energy released kcal/gram	4	9	4

strength. Put simply, their high level of CV training will reduce their already scarce lean muscle supplies as the body turns to its muscle protein for energy.

CARBOHYDRATE

Carbohydrate should constitute 60 per cent of daily diet. Carbohydrate is the body's key fuel source during physical activity. When it's digested, it increases blood sugar levels and provides energy (glucose), through chemical reactions that occur in our muscles.

Carbohydrates are divided into simple types (sugars – also known as monosaccharides) and complex types (fibres and starches – also known as polysaccharides).

Simple carbohydrates contain one or two sugar units in their molecules, while complex carbohydrates contain from 10 units, right up to thousands of units.

Glycogen

Glycogen is a form of carbohydrate. It's produced when our bodies are at rest and carbohydrate travels via the bloodstream to the liver and skeletal muscle where it is converted to and stored as glycogen (muscle fuel). Glycogen is a starch-like substance, made up of numerous glucose molecules. It's very important for exercise. Our glycogen stores are influenced by numerous factors, such as the amount of training we are doing,

rest and carbohydrate consumption. It can only be stored in the body in limited amounts (around 375g) and needs to be continually replenished by carbohydrate consumption after exercise (and during prolonged CV workouts in excess of an hour) to maintain optimum capacity.

In terms of energy potential, our body's average glycogen stores provide 1600–2000kcal – this would release roughly enough energy for one day if we went without food.

Training tip

You should begin your post-workout carbohydrate refuelling as soon as possible after your workout.

Go for 1g of carbohydrate per kg body weight – thus if you weighed 60kg you would need 60g of carbohydrate. You will capitalise on the fact that our bodies replenish their glycogen stores one and a half times more quickly in the two hours after a workout. Go for quick-releasing carbs (those with a high Glycaemic Index *see* page 125).

Two large bananas or 1 litre of a 6 per cent carbohydrate isotonic sports drink will provide you with approximately 50–60g of carbohydrate.

Glycaemic Index – the speed of energy release from carbohydrate

Many foods contain a mixture of simple and complex carbohydrates (*see* page 124), so to measure their immediate energy release they are given a Glycaemic Index (GI) rating. This ranges from 1 to 100. Low GI foods release their energy more slowly than high GI foods. Table 16 identifies the GI ratings of selected foods. It is helpful to understand GI, for everyday use and specific fitness/sports nutrition purposes. This is because it can help control blood sugar levels, thus maintaining energy levels and avoiding over-eating.

The smaller the size of food particles, the more quickly food is digested and the quicker it will release energy – hence the high GI of foods like bread and breakfast cereals.

Table 16 Selected carbohydrates and their GI

Type	GI value	Type	GI value
Sugars		**Fruit and vegetables**	
Glucose	100	Pineapple	66
Sucrose	65	Raisins	66
		Watermelon	72
Bread, rice and pasta		Banana	55
Bread – white	70	Orange	44
Bread – wholemeal	69	Plum	39
Pizza	60	Grapes	46
Rice – brown	76	Apples	38
Rice – white	87	Baked potato	85
		Chips	75
Breakfast cereals		Boiled potato	56
Cornflakes	84	Peas	48
Weetabix	69	Carrots	49
Muesli	56	Broad beans	79
Porridge with water	42		

Table 16 Selected carbohydrates and their GI (cont.)	
Type	**GI value**
Dairy products	
Ice cream	61
Custard	43
Full-fat milk	27
Skimmed milk	32
Pulses	
Red kidney beans	27
Butter beans	31
Soya beans	18
Biscuits and snacks	
Shortbread	64
Rice cakes	85
Tortillas	72
Muesli bar	61
Mars bar	68
Muffin	44
Peanuts	14

Factors to take into account when estimating the energy release of meals:

- Protein and fat reduce GI – slowing the release of energy from food.
- For meals that combine two different GI rated foods in roughly the same quantity – for example, rice and kidney beans – total the GI of the two foods and divide by two. *Example:* rice GI = 87, kidney beans GI = 27, total GI = 114 – therefore the meal's average GI = 57.

Don't emphasise the consumption of high GI foods

High GI foods should be limited in terms of their use throughout the day (apart from assisting training as pre-workout snacks) – this is because they release excessive amounts of the fat storage hormone insulin.

Low GI foods eaten regularly throughout the day will then provide you with a steady supply of energy, which will reduce (normally fat) cravings and help control body weight.

Fibre

Fibre is important for bodily functioning and can only be derived from plant sources. There are two types of fibre:

- Soluble fibre can be partially digested and may help to keep cholesterol figures at healthy levels. Good sources: beans, lentils and oats.
- Insoluble fibre cannot be digested and therefore passes through the body and helps the passage of other food through the gut. This food is stodgy, fills us up, and can reduce over-eating. Good sources: wholegrain bread, breakfast cereals, brown rice and fruit.

Don't be afraid of eating 'properly' after a workout

You'll probably be thinking about those calories that you have 'left' in the gym after a workout. So much so, perhaps, that the thought of eating something straightaway afterwards – which will seemingly cancel out your training – is not high on your agenda. However, eating after a workout can actually have a significant effect on your training and body shaping efforts. Carbohydrate will optimally replenish glycogen stores as noted, and protein will kick-start the re-building of muscle protein that has been broken down by weight training, greatly assisting your muscle and body shaping goals.

Obviously you should not consume too many calories and think you can eat what you like when you are training if you want to lose or balance your weight. *See* page 20 for information on how to calculate your calorific needs and account for your exercise and activity levels.

Do you need to consume carbohydrate drinks during exercise?

If your workout lasts about an hour, then a sports drink – for example, containing carbs – will have little effect on your workout performance and will just add to your total daily calorie intake. Drinking water will be sufficient to maintain hydration. However, if you are a serious CV trainer working out for more than 60 minutes, then carbohydrate can increase your exercise potential and slow down the emptying of your glycogen tank. You'll need to find out what food/drink strategy best suits you.

As a guide, if you weigh 70kg you should consume 30–60g of carbohydrate per hour of exercise depending on workout duration; and if you weigh 60kg, this figure should be 25–50g.

Unrefined foods

Modern food processing and farming methods can reduce the vital vitamin and

Table 17 Food processing, mineral loss and selected foods

Mineral	White flour	Refined sugar	Rice
Chromium	98%	95%	92%
Zinc	78%	88%	54%
Manganese	86%	89%	75%

mineral content of foods below acceptable levels. In Table 17 you'll see why going organic and buying unrefined foods can help to optimise your mineral consumption. White flour loses *98 per cent* of its chromium – a valuable mineral. Always try to opt for unrefined grains.

FAT

Fat should constitute 25–30 per cent of your daily diet. Don't hate fat. It's only bad in high quantities and if too much of the wrong type is consumed. Fat serves numerous essential functions for the body. It is also an energy source – but 1g provides more than twice the calories as carbohydrate and protein. This is why if we don't exercise or watch our consumption, fat will accumulate on our bodies. As has been identified it can be stored on the body as non-essential fat to virtually infinite levels, which is obviously detrimental to health, let alone appearance.

Fat serves crucial functions for the body. As well as providing energy, for example, it is important in terms of hormone metabolism, tissue structure and for the cushioning of other important tissue. And a diet deficient in fat could also lead to a lack of the fat soluble vitamins, A, D and E, and essential fatty acids, the latter of which can negatively affect hormones, influencing the reproductive system.

Cholesterol and fat

Most of us will be aware of cholesterol and may have a negative perception of it. However, cholesterol actually plays a crucial role in our bodies. One of its main functions is to assist the production of numerous hormones. It is in part derived from the food we eat, but is in the main produced in the liver from saturated fats. Too much Low Density Lipoprotein (LDL), or bad cholesterol, is detrimental to (heart) health.

However, it's only bad when its levels in the body are pushed up by factors that include a lack of exercise, obesity, and too great a consumption of saturated fats. LDL builds up in our arteries and restricts the passage of blood, leading to an increase in blood pressure. Unfortunately, it is not until there is a 70 per cent arterial blockage that symptoms reveal themselves.

Ideal cholesterol levels – less than 5.7mmol/1 in the blood
Very high cholesterol level – more than 7.8mmol/1 in the blood

Different types of fat and suggested intakes

Saturated fat

Saturated fat should constitute less than 10 per cent of total fat consumption.

Such fats are found mainly, but not exclusively, in dairy and animal products and are the most 'harmful'. In excess, they can raise low density lipoprotein (LDL) cholesterol (*see* page 128) and lead to heart disease. Examples are butter, cheese and the fat on meat – all are hard at room temperature.

Trans-fatty acids (TFAs) are particularly bad for health and result from the heating, refining and processing of saturated fats to prolong their shelf-life. TFAs are found in fast food and junk food.

Unsaturated fats

- Monounsaturated fats are found in olive oil, nuts and seeds and can reduce LDL cholesterol and its negative effects. These fats are normally liquid at room temperature.
- Polyunsaturated fats are found in most vegetable oils, oily fish, nuts and seeds. They are liquid at room temperature and below. This type of fat can also reduce LDL cholesterol.

It's recommended that around 10 per cent of daily food consumption comes from these fats.

Essential fatty acids – omega-3 and omega-6 series

EFAs cannot be produced in the body and must be provided by food. They serve a crucial hormonal-like function, as they regulate numerous body functions. However, modern food processing methods often results in their nutritional value being significantly reduced.

Omega-3 EFA is found in some nuts and seeds, such as flax and pumpkin seeds, walnuts, soya beans and oily fish, such as sardines, mackerel, salmon, trout and herrings. Common omega-3 fatty acids include alpha linoleic-acid.

Training tip

EFAs, and how they can assist your body shape training

Omega-3 EFAs can:
- Improve oxygen and nutrient transport to cells.
- Reduce the risk of heart attacks.
- Improve the production of aerobic energy.
- Help against strain injuries, as they have anti-inflammatory properties.
- Benefit the immune system, thus reducing susceptibility to illness.
- Increase GH secretion as a consequence of sleep and/or exercise, thus promoting muscle toning and strengthening.

Omega-6 EFAs can:
- Have anti-inflammatory properties.
- Be good for the skin.

Recommendations as to the exact amount of EFAs that active people should consume often conflict. However, as a starting point, aim for 9g of omega-6 and 6g per day of omega-3.

Table 18 The Essential Fatty Acids (EFAs) content of selected foods

Food	Omega-3 per 100g	Omega-6 per 100g
Salmon	3.2	0.7
Walnuts	3.0	3.2
Butter	1.2	1.8
Olive oil	0.6	7.9
Wheat germ	0.5	5.5
Olives	0	1.6

PROTEIN

Protein should constitute 10–15 per cent of your daily diet. When resistance training, muscle protein is broken down and needs to be repaired if the muscle is to get stronger or develop more tone. Protein is crucial for this rebuilding process – that's why it's often referred to as the body's building block.

Protein and amino acids

When protein is digested it's broken down into amino acids; some of these are 'essential' (see Table 19) because they cannot be made in the body, while others are 'non-essential' because they can be made in the body, provided enough of the essential amino acids are present.

Table 19 Essential and non-essential amino acids

Essential amino acids	Non-essential amino acids
Isoleucine	Alanine
Leucine	Arginine
Lysine	Asparagine
Methionine	Aspartic acid
Phenylalanine	Cysteine
Threonine	Glutamic acid
Tryptophan	Glutamine
Valine	Glycine
	Histidine (essential for babies only)
	Proline
	Serine
	Tyrosine

What are the best proteins?

Proteins are given a rating out of 100 that indicates their level of inclusion of all the essential amino acids. This is termed biological value (BV). Proteins with the highest BV are the best at being absorbed into the body and used for growth and repair (*see* Table 20).

Table 20 Protein rating (biological value) of selected proteins

Protein source	Protein rating (biological value) out of 100
Eggs	100
Fish	70
Milk	67
Brown rice	57
Peas	55

Look out for whey proteins in supplements and food products as this is the most quickly absorbed of all proteins.

Turkey, cottage cheese, egg whites, soya beans, semi-skimmed milk and pulses are great low-fat sources of protein.

Vegetarians and protein

If you are a non-meat eater you can obtain your amino acids from plant and vegetable sources, although you will have to be particularly thorough with your nutritional selections. Soya, tofu and quinoa are rich protein sources for vegetarians (and non-vegetarians). This is because they combine high protein content with little fat and are also great sources of carbohydrate.

Micro-nutrients

Many of us are blissfully unaware of the positive effects the micro-nutrients can have on our bodies. Vitamins and minerals can seriously advance your training progress.

MINERALS

Twenty-two mainly metallic minerals make up 4 per cent of our body mass; their main function is to balance and regulate internal chemistry, for example, the maintenance of muscular contractions, the regulation of heart beat and nerve conduction.

Table 21 How much protein do foods contain?

Food	Portion size	Protein (g)
Beef – fillet steak, grilled	105g	31
Chicken breast – grilled, no skin	130g	39
Poached cod	120g	25
Tinned tuna in brine – small can	100g	24
1 glass of skimmed milk	200ml	7
Eggs – size 2	1g	8
Cottage cheese – small carton	112g	15
Peanuts – roasted and salted (handful)	50g	10
Cashew nuts – roasted and salted (handful)	50g	10
Baked beans – small tin	205g	10
Kidney beans – 3 tbs	120g	10
Soya mince – 2 tbs	30g	13

Table 21 How much protein do foods contain? (cont.)

Food	Portion size	Protein (g)
Quorn mince – 4 tbs	110g	12
2 slices wholemeal bread	76g	6
Bowl of boiled pasta	230g	7

VITAMINS

Vitamins are crucial in facilitating energy release from food, but do not produce energy themselves. There are two types:

■ Fat soluble (e.g. A, D, E, K) – stored in the body.
■ Water soluble – cannot be stored in the body and derive from fruit and vegetables.

As with minerals, consuming excess amounts (above their recommended levels/reference nutrient intake – RNI) will not enhance their metabolic contribution.

ANTIOXIDANTS

Antioxidants include the vitamins A, C, E and beta-carotene and the mineral selenium. A diet rich in antioxidants can prevent cellular damage, reduce LDL cholesterol, and defend the body against age-related diseases such as cancer and heart disease.

Antioxidants are especially important when you are training hard, particularly in endurance activities. This is because this type of training can increase free radical cellular damage. What's this? Oxygen fuels the heart and lungs and all bodily processes, including the energy release from food. Unfortunately, this oxygen metabolism can create unstable molecular fragments, which can damage cells if left unchecked. Antioxidant vitamins and minerals (and phytochemicals, which include bioflavonoids; both are contained in brightly coloured fruit and vegetables) can combat this cellular damage. (Note: Recent research has indicated that experienced trainers may suffer less from free-radical damage compared to those starting out on an exercise programme.)

Table 22 Selected vitamins and minerals and their fitness/sports and health benefits and reference nutrient intakes (RNI)

Vitamins/mineral	Function	Reference Nutrient Intake (RNI)	Selected sources
Biotin (B group vitamin)	Assists conversion of food into energy, glycogen manufacture and protein metabolism for muscle building	0.01–0.2mg	Egg yolk, nuts, oats and whole grains, dried mixed fruit
Calcium (mineral)	Assists muscle contraction, hormonal signalling, important for strong bones	700mg	Dairy products, seafood, pulses, flour bread, vegetables
Iron (mineral)	Can assist aerobic exercise by promoting haemoglobin in oxygen-carrying red blood cells. If you lose a lot of blood during your menstrual cycle, then you may need an iron supplement	14.8mg	Liver, red meat, pasta and cereals, green leafy vegetables, eggs, prunes, whole grains and dried fruit

Table 22 Selected vitamins and minerals and their fitness/sports and health benefits and reference nutrient intakes (RNI) (cont.)

Vitamins/mineral	Function	Reference Nutrient Intake (RNI)	Selected sources
Zinc (mineral)	Important for metabolising fats, proteins and carbohydrates	4–7mg	Lean meat and fish, eggs, whole grain cereals, dairy products, whole-grain, wholemeal breads and cereals
Magnesium (mineral)	Boosts energy production and assists muscle contraction, plays a role in blood sugar stabilisation, which assists the balancing of energy levels. Assists formation of new cells	270mg	Green leafy vegetables, fruit, unrefined whole grains and wholegrain cereals, meat and dairy products
Copper (mineral)	Copper assists with collagen (soft tissue) formation and serves as an antioxidant. Assists production of red blood cells	1.2mg	Beef liver, oysters, lamb, peanuts, baked beans, chick peas, wholemeal bread and whole-grain cereals

Vitamins/mineral	Function	Reference Nutrient Intake (RNI)	Selected sources
C (vitamin)	Antioxidant Assists cellular growth and repair. Aids absorption of iron from blood	40mg	Fruit and vegetables, especially, strawberries, oranges, tomatoes, green peppers, baked potatoes

Table 22 Selected vitamins and minerals and their fitness/sports and health benefits and reference nutrient intakes (RNI) (cont.)

Salt

You should restrict your salt consumption to 6g a day. Too much salt can increase your risk of a heart attack. Try to get into the habit of checking food labels for salt content – you may be surprised just how much is 'hidden' in ready meals, take-aways and even so-called 'healthy' meals. In fact about 75 per cent of our salt consumption comes from these sources.

Fluids

It's crucial, whatever your body shape, that you keep hydrated for everyday health and sports reasons. Around 75 per cent of the body is water, and keeping hydrated will ensure the optimisation of all bodily processes.

For everday health, you should aim to drink 2 litres of water a day. This can be derived from 'other' drinks, such as tea. For training or active days, you should aim to consume 1 litre of water for every 1000 calories expended (*see* page 20 for how to calculate your calorific needs).

Water is crucial to optimum body functioning because most of the chemical reactions that occur in our cells need water.

ELECTROLYTES

Electrolytes are mineral salts (sodium, chloride, potassium and magnesium) that are present in bodily fluids. They regulate the fluid balance between different body compartments and the amount of fluid in the bloodstream. As an example, high cellular potassium levels increase the amount of water being pulled across a cell membrane, thus increasing the cell's water content. Sports drinks containing electrolytes have no direct effect on performance; however, sodium encourages your thirst mechanism, making you want to drink more (plain water or sports drinks without electrolytes will not have this effect). This will assist you to optimally hydrate.

Advanced training tip

You should gradually aim to replenish 150 per cent of the fluids lost during exercise. You could work this out by weighing yourself before and after your workout. To calculate how much fluid you have lost and, therefore how much you need to replace, work on the basis that 1 litre of fluid is approximately equivalent to 1kg in weight.

A loss of just 2 per cent (that's 1.5kg if you weigh 75kg) in body weight caused by dehydration could impair CV performance by 10–20 per cent.

Alcohol

You might like the odd glass of wine at the end of the day to relax, that's fine, but be aware that alcohol is calorie dense and will not assist your training.

A glass of red wine contains 85 calories and many pub or restaurant measures are closer to two glasses. A shot of vodka, whisky or gin each contain 55 calories, plus the calorie content of the juice or mixer.

Women can drink up to 2 to 3 units of alcohol a day without a significant health risk, although it is best to have a couple of alcohol-free days per week.

WHAT IS A UNIT?

A unit is half a pint of standard-strength beer, lager or cider, or a pub measure of spirits. A glass of wine is about 2 units and one alcopop is about 1.5 units (Food Standards Agency, www.eatwell.gov.uk).

Supplements

A lot of women ask me about so-called 'miracle' pills, which (according to advertising hype) claim that you'll lose 20lb of body fat in a month! My answer is always the same: there is no miracle product and there are no short cuts to fitness and weight loss. However, there are some very useful supplements that can enhance your workout regime and bring real benefits.

Remember, some supplements can boost your body shaping, fitness and sports performance, but they should only be regarded as accessories to your training.

CREATINE

Creatine has been touted as the 'wonder' sports/fitness supplement and I must admit that most of its claims for improving strength and power performance have been vindicated by sports science research. Creatine is produced naturally in the body from three amino acids. It is found in meat and fish, and is crucial for producing short-lived (anaerobic) energy in muscles (*see* page 16).

How does creatine supplementation work?

Supplementing with creatine boosts your muscles' high energy stores, specifically phosphocreatine (PC). With more of this quick-release energy source available, you'll be able to perform more reps (weights and sprints, for example), which will increase your training adaptation. This could mean more lean muscle mass, boosting your body shaping efforts.

To benefit from creatine it's generally recommended that you need a 'loading phase'. This requires you to take 4 x 5g a day for 5 days and then a maintenance dose of 2g a day for a month. Once the month is up you'll get no further loading benefits and you should cease use for a further month, before starting the process again.

Body shape and why you might want to use creatine

Celery-shaped women could add some curves by providing their muscles with more energy that will enable them to puff up their butts and shape their shoulders through optimised resistance training.

Hourglass shapes training for football or netball will be able to develop greater power and speed by performing successive sprints, with less reduction in performance across efforts, thus boosting their speed potential and match performance.

Are there any problems with using creatine?

Although the majority of research has found no adverse effects from using creatine, older people, pregnant or lactating women, and those with kidney problems, should consult their doctors before starting a supplementation programme.

If you're middle or older aged, then creatine can also be good for you – numerous research studies indicate that it can offset and even increase declining strength, muscle mass and functional mobility.[ii]

Note that the benefits of creatine for enhancing aerobic performance are virtually non-existent.

[ii] See, for example, J Gerontol A Biol Sci Med Sci, 2003, Jan; 58(1): 11-19.

PROTEIN SUPPLEMENTS

Protein supplements have long been used by weight trainers and athletes. As I have indicated, protein is the key component in building, maintaining and repairing muscle.

You should aim for 1.4–1.6g of protein per kilogram of body weight and resistance train if you want to build more shapely curves. Protein supplements can be beneficial for vegetarians and for women whose diet is low in protein.

Recent research has highlighted the importance of consuming protein prior to resistance training in order to prime muscle for positive adaptation. It has been well known for quite some time that supplementing post-exercise will increase the rate of protein synthesis and speed up the recovery and the growth of new, stronger muscle tissue.

Are there problems with taking in too much protein?

Too much protein (and too little carbohydrate) can lead to digestive problems, nausea, bad breath, osteoporosis and a lack of essential micro-nutrients being absorbed into the body.

Protein versus carbohydrate

When it comes to the 'protein versus carbohydrate diet and supplement question', the answer is you need both. Carbohydrate is the body's key energy macro-nutrient. You need it to keep your body's energy stores supplied and fuel your training. Go for quick-releasing carb (high GI) supplements, such as energy bars/drinks prior to and during workouts (particularly CV ones that last in excess of an hour) and slower-releasing (low GI) meals and snacks throughout your day to keep your energy levels balanced, and to avoid cravings and fat accumulation (see Glycaemic Index, page 125).

WEIGHT GAIN SUPPLEMENTS

Very few women will believe that they need a weight gain supplement. However, if you are a celery shape or a slighter hourglass and you are after increased muscle for aesthetic or sports performance (and are of any body shape and in very hard training) then these supplements can be of use. This is because you will need to considerably increase your calorie consumption in order to provide energy and sufficient muscle building protein and energy-providing carbs. Your 'normal' calorific intake may be insufficient to do this. In this instance, a specific supplement, such as a 'weight gain' one, can be useful – due to the hundreds of additional calories it will supply. These usually combine whey protein with good, quick-energy releasing carbs. Some also contain specific fats (essential fatty acids – see page 129), which are calorie dense, valuable for numerous body functions, good energy suppliers and less likely to be turned into body fat.

The problem with not eating enough

Women are particularly susceptible to under-eating when in training and also in everyday life. Supplements should never replace meals. Not only will under-eating compromise your training and your adaptation, it could also compromise your health, as your reduced calories may result in insufficient micro-nutrient absorption. You also run the risk of metabolic slowdown.

Advanced exercisers could need in excess of 3000 calories a day. The average UK diet provides only 5mg of iron per 1000 calories. As the RDA is 14.8mg per day and active women often consume less than 2000kcal a day, it becomes apparent just how important optimum calorie consumption and/or a supplement programme is for ensuring optimum iron intake.

Supplements will only get you so far; they should not be seen as substitutes for a carefully tailored healthy diet, specific to your progressive training plan.

MULTIVITAMINS/MULTIMINERALS

If you are not getting your 5 a day of fruit and vegetables, then a multivitamin/multimineral supplement can be particularly useful – although you should always try to get your nutrients from food sources. A good multivitamin should contain vitamins and minerals such as vitamin C, the B group, zinc, calcium and iron.

FAT BURNERS

This may be one supplement that will grab your attention! However, before you buy a supply from the healthshop shelves, read on. Fat burning products are designed to elevate your body's metabolic rate and mobilise fat as an energy source. Many contain the stimulants caffeine and guarana. Some research has discovered the presence of International Olympic Committee banned drugs such as ephedrine in some claimed 'natural' products. I therefore recommend that fat burning products should be avoided – regular training and a balanced diet will up your metabolic rate and burn fat naturally. As I've previously pointed out, regular training can elevate metabolic rate by as much as 20 per cent.

CHECK YOUR SUPPLEMENTS

You should always check the supplement product labelling and buy from a reputable supplier. Most products are designed for those with lactose intolerance. If in doubt, consult a health professional or nutritionist.

SUPPLEMENTS DESIGNED TO MAINTAIN YOUR BODY'S JOINTS

Recently there has been a growth in the promotion of joint-health supplements, often containing glucosamine sulphate or chondroitin. Taking these can be beneficial for all women in regular training.

Glucosamine is a natural non-toxic compound found in the body. It is used in the manufacture of very large molecules found in joint cartilage; basically, these hold on to water, rather like a sponge, and in doing so provide cushioning for joints. A number of reputable surveys have indicated that it can prevent knee joint narrowing (and the further development of arthritis) and reduce pain.[iii]

Chondroitin is another naturally occurring body compound. Like glucosamine, it is involved in the repair and maintenance of joints. Research is more limited at present, compared to that done on glucosamine, although those surveys that exist indicate that chondroitin can reduce joint pain, increase mobility and reduce inflammation.

To build up working chondroitin and glucosamine levels in the body, try a combined supplement, ingesting 1500mg daily. The ratio should be 1000g of glucosamine to 500g of chondroitin.

As with other supplements, it is advisable to check with your doctor before taking glucosamine and chondroitin. For example, people with diabetes should check their blood sugar levels more frequently when taking glucosamine.

[iii] *Lancet*, 2001, 357: 251–6.

BASIC NUTRITION PROGRAMMES FOR SELECTED TRAINING GOALS AND BODY SHAPES

It would be beyond the scope of this book to provide detailed eating plans for 'celeries', 'hourglasses', 'apples' and 'pears'. I have therefore decided to focus on some common body shape training goals, notably fat loss and body shaping. By studying their contents you will be able to pull out the key information that applies to you and construct a relevant eating programme.

Goal: body shaping by increasing leanness

Key workout task: If you are looking to fill out your jeans in the right places, for example, then increasing your lean muscle will be high on your agenda. In terms of workouts, weight training will be key and your priority will be to stimulate muscle growth via high-intensity medium/heavy weight training (CV work should be kept to a minimum, but not overlooked, as it is very important for general health).

Key nutrition task: In terms of nutrition you'll want to ensure optimum protein consumption and timing to 'grow' more shapely muscles and ensure carbohydrate consumption maintains your energy levels and replenishes glycogen levels. You'll also need to consume healthy fat, to permit nutrient balance and to avoid unwanted fat accumulation.

Energy balance: Positive – up to 20 per cent more calories may be needed than those required to balance energy needs. You need to be training regularly 3–4 times a week.

Body shape concerns (where applicable)
'Celery'. Of all body shapes, 'celeries' will have to ensure optimum nutrition to shape muscle, due to their already reduced muscle mass and higher metabolic rates

Overweight 'apple' or 'pear'. If you are overweight and want bigger muscles, then you are probably best suited to following a training programme that involves a high CV content initially to reduce body weight, before progressing to a more focused resistance programme. You'll have to remove fat before revealing your muscles. Once you have reduced, you can then begin to target your lean mass more specifically with an intense resistance training routine. If you feel that you want to lose more realistic weight while building more muscle, you could reduce your calorie consumption by 15 per cent, 3–4 days a week on the days you don't train. On the days you *do* train, you'll need to ensure you create a positive energy balance by around 10 per cent.

HOW MUCH LEAN MUSCLE GAIN CAN YOU EXPECT?

The majority of women can expect to gain 0.25–0.75kg of muscle per month as a result of a regular (two to three times a week) weight training programme. Regardless of your age, you can increase your strength and muscle mass.

Training tip

'Celeries' could benefit from consuming denser forms of carbohydrate, such as dried fruit and honey, due to their faster metabolisms. 'Apples', 'pears' and overweight hourglass figures should go for natural fibre-rich carbohydrates, which are more filling.

Goal: fat/weight loss

With the ever-growing obesity epidemic, and emphasis on the female body form in the media, it is more than likely that the majority of women reading this book will be concerned with losing weight rather than building themselves up.

Key workout task: Emphasis on X-training – that's combining CV and resistance workouts to stimulate lean muscle mass, burn fat and increase everyday metabolic rate.

Key nutrition task: As with increasing lean muscle, the nutritional aim must be to ensure optimum protein consumption and timing to increase lean muscle mass and boost metabolic rate. Carbohydrate consumption must maintain energy and replenish glycogen levels to optimise training readiness; however, it must be controlled to prevent a positive energy balance and weight gain. Healthy fat consumption is equally important – reduce its daily consumption percentage to 25 per cent, increasing protein accordingly.

Desired energy balance: Negative. Use the guide on page 20 to work out your estimated calorific needs. Note that calorie reduction should be controlled and carefully implemented – avoid drastic cuts, which could result in metabolic slow down – see page 20.

Try this: On non-training days, under-eat by 200–300 calories and maintain a balanced energy balance on your training days. After a while you may find that your lean muscle mass is declining (after shaping up). If this is the case, you will have to increase your calorific consumption to maintain your lean muscle. The best way to do this would be to create a positive energy balance on the days you train by 300–600 calories (depending on the intensity of your workouts). (Note: On training days and non-training days you should maintain the same amount of protein consumption: 1.4–1.6g per kilogram of body weight.)

WEIGHT LOSS TIPS

- Don't reduce your daily calorie consumption by more than 15 per cent. It might be tempting to cut back more significantly on calories than this. However, doing so runs the risk of slowing down your metabolic rate as your body hangs on to the fewer calories it gets (this is sometimes known as 'famine/starvation mode'). Huge calorie cuts can reduce metabolic rate by as much as 45 per cent. Insufficient calorific consumption will also significantly impair our workout (and everyday activity) performance.
- Create a negative energy balance. As there are 3500 calories in 0.45kg (1 lb) of body weight, a 300-calorie daily deficit would theoretically get rid of this in approximately 12 days. This negative balance can be achieved by calorie restriction and increased calorie expenditure through exercise. Note that in reality your body type/body shape, age and genetic disposition will affect your weight loss potential. Note also that if you are in regular training you need to ensure sufficient calorie consumption to fuel your training, therefore it is not recommended to create a negative energy balance on a daily basis.
- Don't 'yo-yo' diet. Rapid increases and decreases in calorie consumption can throw your metabolism off-line and so increase the risk of metabolic slow-down.
- Continually monitor your workouts and the resulting increase in your fitness as it affects calories burning. As your fitness improves, your body will become more exercise efficient. This means that you'll have to increase your workout intensity to continue to burn as many or more calories than you did when you first started out. (Note: For safe training progression, do not increase intensity and duration at the same time.)
- Don't become preoccupied with where the calories you burn during your workouts come from (i.e. fat or carbohydrate). As I have indicated, what really matters is total exercise calorie burn.
- Don't believe that a specific 'fat burning zone' exists. All exercise options, both CV and resistance, can burn fat and help you achieve the body you desire.
- Don't skip meals; calculate your calorific needs and eat frequently (five or six times) during the day. Research indicates that those who eat the most and train the most are usually the leanest and fittest.

What to actually eat!

Women tend to have a better idea about food content and what to eat than guys, but if you are starting a new eating plan for life, or your current diet is causing you to gain weight, you may want some useful pointers. I have therefore given you the macro-nutrient content of certain healthy foods, to help you plan your meals (Table 23). I have also provided other reference sources where you can find out about more foods. You'll also see that the meals are simple to prepare!

Table 23 Macro-nutrient content of healthy foods

Breakfast

Food	Kcal	Protein (g)	Carbohydrate (g)	Fat (g)
1 cup (60g) porridge oats	241	7	44	5
300ml skimmed milk	99	10	15	0
1 tbs (30g) raisins	82	1	21	0
2 slices wholegrain toast	174	7	34	2
2 tsp olive oil spread	57	0	0	6
2 scrambled or poached eggs	160	14	0	12
3 Shredded Wheat	228	7	48	2
1 bowl muesli (60g)	220	6	40	5
4 heaped tsp honey	173	0	46	0
Glass of orange juice	72	1	18	0
1 tbs peanut butter	242	10	2	21
Low-fat fruit yoghurt (150g)	135	6	27	1
Egg large (raw)	74	6	Trace	5

Table 23 Macro-nutrient content of healthy foods (cont.)

Mid-morning snacks

Food	Kcal	Protein (g)	Carbohydrate (g)	Fat (g)
2 bananas	190	2	46	1
2 energy bars (66g)	309	7	40	15
2 apples	94	1	24	0
Peanut butter sandwich with 2 slices wholegrain bread and 1 tbs of peanut butter	174 242	7 10	34 3	2 21

Lunch/dinner

1 large baked potato (225g) with olive oil spread, tuna in brine (100g), salad (125g)	505	34	71	10
1 wholegrain pitta, 2 tbs olive oil spread, 2 slices turkey (70g), 1 bowl salad (125g)	343	25	36	12

Table 23 Macro-nutrient content of healthy foods (cont.)				
Food	**Kcal**	**Protein (g)**	**Carbohydrate (g)**	**Fat (g)**
Pasta salad, 2 tbs tuna in brine, large handful chopped peppers, 1 tbs olive oil dressing	563	33	82	14
Baked potato as above, plus chicken (70g), sweetcorn (125g), salad (125g), 1 tbs olive oil dressing	373	35	106	15
Large portion grilled chicken (120g), pasta (85g, uncooked), 1 tbs olive oil, large portion broccoli and carrots, pasta sauce	645	52	75	19
Grilled turkey breast (100g), noodles (100g, uncooked), cauliflower	517	37	78	9
Grilled white fish (175g), large sweet potato, carrots, courgettes	549	45	90	3
Grilled salmon (175g), brown rice (115g), spinach	743	46	94	23

Table 23 Macro-nutrient content of healthy foods (cont.)				
Food	Kcal	Protein (g)	Carbohydrate (g)	Fat (g)
Sirloin steak grilled (90g)	206	30	0	9
Canned light tuna	116	26	0	1
Ham, extra lean sliced (90g)	131	20	1	5
Cod (90g)	105	23	0	1
Lunch/dinner				
Protein bar/cereal bar (33g)	154	3	20	7
Meal replacement supplement (1 serving)	174	18	26	0
Orange	59	2	14	0
Low-fat yoghurt (150g)	135	6	27	1
2 bananas	190	2	46	1

Note: There are approximately twice as many calories in fat compared to protein and carbohydrate (approximately 9:4).

Source: Adapted from Bean, A., *The Complete Guide to Sports Nutrition* (4th edition).

Understanding food labels

Learning how to read and understand food labels can be very empowering when it comes to your health and nutrition, and I recommend checking out contents wherever possible. Try to avoid artificial flavours, colours, E numbers and too many preservatives. I believe that a diet consisting of foods as close to their natural state as possible is the best thing for your health and body shape. Whoever said 'You are what you eat' was spot on.

There is a legal requirement for the content of foods to be listed on the packaging in the UK (this means that foods sold loose are currently exempt from labelling).

Key food labelling requirements:

- The content of the product must be clearly listed (many foods have names that are irrelevant to the product).
- The content has to be clear to the user, but this *still* might not be unless you apply your grey matter! For example, 'fruit flavoured yoghurt' can contain artificial flavourings, while 'fruit yoghurt' must contain fruit.
- The food processing method used (if any) must be listed; for example, smoked salmon, roasted peanuts.
- The weight (accurate to within a couple of grams) must be stated.
- Ingredients are listed in weight order – this must include water and any additives.
- Genetically modified foods must state they are GM.
- Storage and preparation instructions must be provided.

Interestingly, nutrition information does not have to be displayed, unless the manufacturer makes a specific nutritional claim. When this claim is made, the information relating to it must be presented as follows:

- Energy value provided in kilojoules (kJ) and kilocalories (kcal).
- Macro-nutrient content (protein, carbohydrate and fat) listed in grams (g).
- The manufacturer may also choose to list the amounts of sugars, saturates, fibre and sodium.
- Information on other constituents, such as the type of fat in the product, can be listed. (It is crucial to look for products that list all their ingredients. This will enable you to reduce those that are harmful to health – in large quantities, saturated and

especially trans-fatty acids for example, *see* page 129.)

- If the vitamin and mineral content of the product is listed as a percentage, this is usually termed the Recommended Daily Allowance (RDA). RDAs are part of European Union legislation and represent an averaging of the RDA opinion from the EU member countries and their citizens.

GUIDELINE DAILY AMOUNTS

Some products may also state guideline daily amounts. These provide an estimate of the number of calories men and women aged between 19 and 50 of 'normal weight and fitness' require. This figure is 2000kcal for women. These figures should be viewed with caution as they do not account for specific body shapes and training status, for example.

Table 24 Portion sizes for your 5-a-day		
Fruit	Apple, pear, banana, orange	1
	Berries (strawberries, raspberries, blackberries, grapes)	80g (1 cup full)
	Melon, pineapple	Large slice
	Tinned fruit (any type)	⅓ of a 400g tin
	Fruit juice	Glass (150ml)
	Dried fruit	1 tbsp
Vegetables	Carrots/courgettes	1 large
	Broccoli	2 spears
	Mixed salad	Dessert bowl
	Tomato	2
	Cucumber	3 slices

WHAT IS A PORTION (SELECTED FRUIT AND VEGETABLES)?

Further advice on understanding units of food measurement

A gram is about the weight of a Smartie. Apart from calcium and potassium, the amounts of each nutrient required by the body each day are much less than a gram, so other, much smaller, units are used.

- The milligram – is abbreviated mg and is one-thousandth of a gram. There are 1000mg in a gram.
- The microgram – is abbreviated mcg and is one-millionth of a gram. There are 1000mcg in each milligram.
- The International Unit – is abbreviated IU. It is sometimes used instead of mg or mcg for some of the vitamins such as A, D and E where there is more than one form of a vitamin. International Units express the biological activity that different forms of a vitamin exhibit.
- UK Reference Nutrient Intake – the daily amount deemed adequate to prevent deficiencies in 97.5 per cent of the UK population; this can also be displayed on food and is used by nutritionists.

CONCLUSION

You are already one step closer to a healthier, fitter you! By reading this book you have made a positive step in the right direction, and sometimes that first step is the hardest step to take. Now you need to move forward and make small, positive steps each day. Remember that you need to set goals and have a new balanced approach to food and exercise. Try not to be impatient as your body shape will not change overnight, but rest assured that with a positive mind-set and a realistic, balanced programme, you can change your body for good. Try to lead an active life and embrace every opportunity to move your body – walk to the shops and carry your goods home in a backpack, cycle to the train station in the morning, or walk the children to school. Many of my clients mention the positive effects that these life changes have on their outlook, their stress levels and their happiness as well as their body shapes. Be kind to yourself! Do not set unachievable goals (remember your body type) and don't punish yourself for failing – set a long-term goal, with several short-term achievable goals to lead the way. You'll get there. Remember that exercise should be fun, and the positive effects from your efforts will go way beyond a slimmer waistline.

So, good luck with your healthier lifestyle, stay positive and enjoy your journey!

INDEX